Practice questions in Psychopharmacology

Volume 1

Dr. Srikanth Sajja
Humber NHS Foundation Trust
Hull, UK

Professor Ann M Mortimer
Foundation Chair
Head of the Department of Psychiatry
University of Hull
Hull, UK

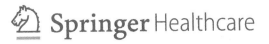
Springer Healthcare

Published by Springer Healthcare Ltd, 236 Gray's Inn Road, London, WC1X 8HB, UK.

www.springerhealthcare.com

British Library Cataloguing-in-Publication Data.

A catalogue record for this book is available from the British Library.

Although every effort has been made to ensure that drug doses and other information are presented accurately in this publication, the ultimate responsibility rests with the prescribing physician. Neither the publisher nor the authors can be held responsible for errors or for any consequences arising from the use of the information contained herein. Any product mentioned in this publication should be used in accordance with the prescribing information prepared by the manufacturers. No claims or endorsements are made for any drug or compound at present under clinical investigation.

Cover photo by Srikanth Sajja LRPS.

Project editor: Hannah Cole
Designer: Joe Harvey
Artworker: Sissan Mollerfors
Production: Marina Maher

This book is a welcome addition to currently available resources in psychopharmacology for trainees. Questions on psychopharmacology (including basic and clinical psychopharmacology and therapeutics) are common topics in the psychiatry field and many trainees have difficulties with them.

Dr Sajja is to be commended for producing an excellent series of relevant questions and has used an extensive bibliography to generate topics that will be both a useful test of progression as well as a memory aid and primer.

I often think the best answer to any psychopharmacology question is "I'll look it up!" Given the size of the Data Sheet Compendium and other psychopharmacology volumes, this is a sensible strategy for clinical management. However, this is not a recourse that one can use in an exam, although this book should help considerably with most major examinations in this field.

Professor I. Nicol Ferrier
Academic Psychiatry, Institute of Neuroscience
Newcastle General Hospital
Newcastle, UK

Acknowledgements

I would very much like to thank Professor Ann Mortimer for making valuable suggestions and being a source of inspiration by joining me as a co-author.

I am grateful to the post-graduate trainees, my colleagues and leading academicians in psychopharmacology for their useful feedback and encouragement.

I also thank Dr Dave Armstrong for his assistance in preparing some questions related to alcohol and drug abuse.

I am deeply indebted to Professor Nicol Ferrier for kindly providing the Foreword to the book.

I gratefully acknowledge the encouragement received from my parents and the patience shown by my wife and my daughter during the completion of this task.

I also thank my secretary Sheila Jenkinson for preparing this manuscript in time.

My special thanks to Hannah Cole, my publisher, for her guidance and support.

And finally, I owe my gratitude to my patients for making me constantly think and update my knowledge in this wonderful and challenging field of psychopharmacology.

Srikanth Sajja
2011

Preface

Psychopharmacology is a fascinating and exciting speciality that is constantly undergoing new and rapid scientific developments with clinical applications. The aim of this book is to provide practice questions in psychopharmacology to facilitate learning and revision. It consists of 2600 questions in the form of 'True/False Individual Statements, Extended Matching Items and Best of Five' formats, organised in 52 papers in two volumes.

Every attempt has been made to cover all relevant topics in psychopharmacology, addressing both knowledge and clinical competency related to the speciality. Resources used to prepare the questions are provided in the 'reading list' at the end, giving access to extensive cross-references.

This book will be a useful means of self-assessment for both trainees and practitioners in the fields of psychiatry, neurology, pharmacology, psychiatric pharmacy and general medicine.

Srikanth Sajja
2011

Topics covered

Development of Psychotropic Drugs

Research Methodology for Drug Trials

Receptors

Pharmacokinetics

Pharmacodynamics

Pharmacogenetics

Anxiolytics, hypnotics

Antipsychotic drugs

Mood Stabilisers

Antidepressant Drugs

Antimuscarinic Drugs

Antiepileptic Drugs

Drugs Used in Movement Disorders

Drugs Used in Substance Dependence

Antidementia Drugs

Adverse Reactions

Drug Interactions

Pharmacological Treatment of Psychiatric Disorders

Psychopharmacology of Children

Psychopharmocology of Elderly

Psychopharmacology of Women

Psychotropic Drugs in Special Patient Groups

New Drugs

Pharmacoeconomics

Psycho Socio Cultural Aspects of Psychopharmacology

Paper 1

	True	False
1. Norquetiapine mediates the inhibition of noradrenaline transporter.	☐	☐
2. Ion channels are exclusively voltage-gated.	☐	☐
3. Upregulation of receptors means an increase in neurotransmitter receptor synthesis.	☐	☐
4. Antagonists block the actions of agonists but not inverse agonists.	☐	☐
5. Inverse agonists block the actions of agonists.	☐	☐
6. The 5-HT3 receptor is a G-protein-linked receptor.	☐	☐
7. Kinases and phosphatases are third messengers.	☐	☐
8. Concomitant use of fluoxetine and tramadol can cause serotonin syndrome.	☐	☐
9. Aripiprazole is an antagonist at postsynaptic D2 receptors and an agonist at presynaptic dopamine autoreceptors.	☐	☐
10. Nemonapride is a potent 5-HT2A receptor antagonist.	☐	☐
11. Tianeptine is a serotonin reuptake inhibitor.	☐	☐
12. Buspirone shows cross-tolerance with the benzodiazepines.	☐	☐
13. Agomelatin reduces the discontinuation symptoms of SSRIs.	☐	☐
14. Long-term use of paroxetine is associated with weight gain.	☐	☐
15. Social phobia is a contra-indication for β-adrenergic receptor antagonists.	☐	☐
16. Propranalol is effective in the treatment of neuroleptic-induced acute dystonia.	☐	☐
17. Bradycardia and hypotension are the most common adverse effects of β-adrenergic receptor antagonists.	☐	☐
18. Amantadine is metabolised by oxidation.	☐	☐
19. Trihexyphenidyl is associated with abuse potential.	☐	☐
20. Features of anticholinergic intoxication include delirium, seizures, hallucinations and supraventricular tachycardia.	☐	☐
21. Physostigmine is an inhibitor of anticholinesterase.	☐	☐
22. The CYP2D6 gene is located on the long arm of chromosome 10.	☐	☐
23. Nociceptin is an opioid antagonist.	☐	☐
24. Substance P acts at NK1 receptor.	☐	☐
25. Lorazepam is metabolised by oxidation.	☐	☐
26. Zolpidem and zaliplon are GABA-A positive allosteric modulators.	☐	☐
27. Acetycholine is a neurotransmitter at all preganglionic sympathetic nerve terminals.	☐	☐

28. D3 receptor is a D1-like receptor. ☐ ☐

29. GABA-B receptors are metabotropic and coupled to Ca2+ and K+ channels. ☐ ☐

30. NMDA receptors are not inotropic glutamate receptors. ☐ ☐

31. Nitrazepam and temazepam do not form active metabolites. ☐ ☐

32. Inhibitory amino acid neurotransmitters open Na+ channels. ☐ ☐

33. Tremor is the most common feature of abrupt LSD withdrawal. ☐ ☐

34. Sodium valproate induces the metabolism of phenytoin and carbamazepine. ☐ ☐

35. Vigabatrin is an irreversible inhibitor of glutamic acid decarboxylase (GAD). ☐ ☐

36. Central cholecystokinin receptor agonists are potent panicogenic agents. ☐ ☐

37. Fluvoxamine inhibits the degradation of clozapine. ☐ ☐

38. Female gender and older age are known risk factors for neuroleptic-induced acute dystonia. ☐ ☐

39. Leuprolide is a leutinizing hormone – releasing hormone (LHRH) antagonist. ☐ ☐

40. Galantamine is a carbamate derivative. ☐ ☐

41. Increased levels of plasma branched chain amino acids (BCAA) is associated with a reduction of the symptoms of tardive dyskinesia. ☐ ☐

42. The risk of seizure is not increased by clozapine. ☐ ☐

43. Sertraline is contraindicated in the treatment of depression post-MI. ☐ ☐

44. Neuroleptic malignant syndrome occurs late in the course of treatment. ☐ ☐

45. Clozapine shows larger ratio between FOS protein expression in the medial prefrontal cortex and in the dorsdolateral striatum than measured for haloperidol. ☐ ☐

46. In general partial agonists have greater safety profiles than full agonists. ☐ ☐

47. Memantine hydrochloride is a partial agonist at NMDA receptor. ☐ ☐

48. Coexistence of neurotransmitters and peptides proves that Dale's law does not always apply. ☐ ☐

49. Peptides are of lower molecular weight than neurotransmitters. ☐ ☐

50. Second messenger mediated mechanisms are faster than voltage-dependent mechanisms. ☐ ☐

Paper 1

1. **Norquetiapine mediates the inhibition of noradrenaline transporter.**

Ans. **True.**

2. **Ion channels are exclusively voltage-gated.**

Ans. **False.** They can be either (ligand-gated (Cl) or voltage-gated (Na,K,Ca).

3. **Upregulation of receptors means an increase in neurotransmitter receptor synthesis.**

Ans. **True.**

4. **Antagonists block the actions of agonists but not inverse agonists.**

Ans. **False.** Antagonists block the actions of both agonists, and inverse agonists.

5. **Inverse agonists block the actions of agonists.**

Ans. **False.** Inverse agonists do not block the actions of agonists, but do the opposite of the agonists.

6. **The 5-HT3 receptor is a G-protein-linked receptor.**

Ans. **False.** 5-HT3 receptor is a ligand-gated ion channel, whereas all the other serotonin receptors are G-protein-linked.

7. **Kinases and phosphatases are third messengers.**

Ans. **True.**

8. **Concomitant use of fluoxetine and tramadol can cause serotonin syndrome.**

Ans. **True.**

9. **Aripiprazole is an antagonist at postsynaptic D2 receptors and an agonist at presynaptic dopamine autoreceptors.**

Ans. **True.**

10. **Nemonapride is a potent 5-HT2A receptor antagonist.**

Ans. **False.** Nemonapride is a benzomide derivative and a potent and highly selective D2 receptor antagonist.

11. **Tianeptine is a serotonin reuptake inhibitor.**

Ans. **False.** Tianeptine is a serotonin uptake enhancer that acts as an antidepressant.

12. **Buspirone shows cross-tolerance with the benzodiazepines.**

Ans. **False.** Buspirone is a non-benzodiazepine anxiolytic that is a 5-HT1a agonist.

13. **Agomelatin reduces the discontinuation symptoms of SSRIs.**

Ans. **False.**

14. **Long-term use of paroxetine is associated with weight gain.**

Ans. **True.**

15. **Social phobia is a contra-indication for β-adrenergic receptor antagonists.**

Ans. **False.** β-Adrenergic receptor antagonists are effective in social phobia.

16. **Propranalol is effective in the treatment of neuroleptic-induced acute dystonia.**

Ans. **False.**

17. **Bradycardia and hypotension are the most common adverse effects of β-adrenergic receptor antagonists.**

Ans. **True.**

18. **Amantadine is metabolised by oxidation.**

Ans. **False.** Amantadine is excreted unmetabolised in urine.

19. **Trihexyphenidyl is associated with abuse potential.**

Ans. **True.** Trihexyphenidyl has stimulating properties.

20. **Features of anticholinergic intoxication include delirium, seizures, hallucinations and supraventricular tachycardia.**

Ans. **True.**

21. **Physostigmine is an inhibitor of anticholinesterase.**

Ans. **True.**

22. **The CYP2D6 gene is located on the long arm of chromosome 10.**

Ans. **False.** Chromosome 22 at 22q13.1.

23. **Nociceptin is an opioid antagonist.**

Ans. **False.** Nociceptin is an endogenous orphan opioid receptor (ORL1) agonist. Opioid receptors are divided into µ1, µ2, δ1, δ2, κ1, κ2, κ3 and ORL1.

24. **Substance P acts at NK1 receptor.**

Ans. **True.** Substance P is a neuropeptide and acts at NK, tachytonin receptor. (NK2 and NK3 are the other two types).

25. **Lorazepam is metabolised by oxidation.**

Ans. **False.** Lorazepam is conjugated to form lorazepam glucoronide.

26. **Zolpidem and zaliplon are GABA-A positive allosteric modulators.**

Ans. **True.**

27. **Acetycholine is a neurotransmitter at all preganglionic sympathetic nerve terminals.**

Ans. **True.**

28. **D3 receptor is a D1-like receptor.**

Ans. **False.** D1 and D5 are D1-like and D2, D3 and D4 are D2-like receptors.

29. **GABA-B receptors are metabotropic and coupled to Ca2+ and K+ channels.**

Ans. **True.**

30. **NMDA receptors are not inotropic glutamate receptors.**

Ans. **False.** Inotropic glutamate receptors are subdivided into NMDA (N-Methyl-D-aspartic acid), AMPA (Amino-3OH-5-Methyl-4-isoxazole propionic acid) and Kainate receptors.

31. **Nitrazepam and temazepam do not form active metabolites.**

Ans. **True.**

32. **Inhibitory amino acid neurotransmitters open Na+ channels.**

Ans. **False.** Inhibitory amino acid neurotransmitters open Cl- channels causing hyperpolarisation. Excitatory amino acid transmitters open Na+ channels causing depolarisation.

33. **Tremor is the most common feature of abrupt LSD withdrawal.**

Ans. **False.** There are no physical or psychological symptoms on abrupt LSD withdrawal.

34. **Sodium valproate induces the metabolism of phenytoin and carbamazepine.**

Ans. **False.** Sodium valproate inhibits the metabolism of pheytoin

35. **Vigabatrin is an irreversible inhibitor of glutamic acid decarboxylase (GAD).**

Ans. **False.** Vigabatin is an irreversible inhibitor of GABA transaminase.

36. **Central cholecystokinin receptor agonists are potent panicogenic agents.**

Ans. **True.**

37. **Fluvoxamine inhibits the degradation of clozapine.**

Ans. **True.** By inhibiting CYP1A2 and CYP3A4.

38. **Female gender and older age are known risk factors for neuroleptic-induced acute dystonia.**

Ans. **False.** Male gender and younger age are risk factors for neuropletic induced acute dystonia.

39. **Leuprolide is a leutinizing hormone – releasing hormone (LHRH) antagonist.**

Ans. **False.** Leuprolide is a LHRH agonist. It acts as a sex-drive depressant.

40. **Galantamine is a carbamate derivative.**

Ans. **False.** Galantamine is a phenanthrene alkaloid.

41. **Increased levels of plasma branched chain amino acids (BCAA) is associated with a reduction of the symptoms of tardive dyskinesia.**

Ans. **True.** Ingestion of BCAA reduces plasma levels of phenylalanine and its availability to the brain.

42. **The risk of seizure is not increased by clozapine.**

Ans. **False.** Clozapine increases the risk of seizure by 3.5%

43. **Sertraline is contraindicated in the treatment of depression post-MI.**

Ans. **False.** Recommended.

44. **Neuroleptic malignant syndrome occurs late in the course of treatment.**

Ans. **False.** Neuroleptic malignant syndrome occurs early in the course of treatmemt.

45. **Clozapine shows larger ratio between FOS protein expression in the medial prefrontal cortex and in the dorsdolateral striatum than measured for haloperidol.**

Ans. **True.**

46. **In general partial agonists have greater safety profiles than full agonists.**

Ans. **True.**

47. **Memantine hydrochloride is a partial agonist at NMDA receptor.**

Ans. **False.** Memantine hydrochloride is an NMDA antagonist used for the treatment of moderately severe to severe Alzheimer's disease.

48. **Coexistence of neurotransmitters and peptides proves that Dale's law does not always apply.**

Ans. **True.**

49. **Peptides are of lower molecular weight than neurotransmitters.**

Ans. **False.** Neurotransmitters are of lower molecular weight than peptides.

50. **Second messenger mediated mechanisms are faster than voltage-dependent mechanisms.**

Ans. **False.** Second messenger mediated mechanisms are faster than voltage dependent mechanisms.

Paper 2

		True	False
1.	Tubocurarine is a nicotinic receptor antagonist.	☐	☐
2.	In a dose-response curve ED50 represents the dose which elicits 50% of the maximal response and Emax represents the dose which elicits maximum response.	☐	☐
3.	IC50 represents the concentration of antagonist needed to displace the ligand from 50% of the available receptors.	☐	☐
4.	Co-administration of tryptophan and an MAOI should be avoided.	☐	☐
5.	Mianserin causes the blockade of alpha 2 adrenoceptors and 5-HT2 receptors.	☐	☐
6.	d-serine is an NMDA receptor antagonist.	☐	☐
7.	d-cycloserine is a partial agonist at the NMDA receptor glycine site.	☐	☐
8.	In some trials, sigma receptor antagonists have shown an antipsychotic effect.	☐	☐
9.	GABA-A receptor agonists might be of some use as adjuvants in the treatment of schizophrenia.	☐	☐
10.	Omega-3 fatty acids are shown to be increased in the neuronal membranes of schizophrenic patients.	☐	☐
11.	Antidepressant drugs are not associated with tolerance and craving.	☐	☐
12.	Iloperidone is a new antipsychotic with very high affinity for alpha-2 adrenoceptors.	☐	☐
13.	Methylphenidate is a controlled class B drug in the UK used in the treatment of attention deficit hyperactivity disorder.	☐	☐
14.	More than 90% of unchanged aripiprazole is renally excreted.	☐	☐
15.	In the treatment of drug addiction, diamorphine can be prescribed in the UK without a special licence.	☐	☐
16.	Coproxamol overdosage presents with pinpoint pupils and respiratory depression.	☐	☐
17.	Neostigmine reverses the action of the depolarising muscle relaxant suxamethonium.	☐	☐
18.	Anticholinesterases such as neostigmine reverse the effects of the non- depolarised muscle relaxant drugs.	☐	☐
19.	Naloxone reverses opioid-induced respiratory depression.	☐	☐
20.	Dantrolene worsens the symptoms of malignant hyperthermia.	☐	☐
21.	Active metabolites are rarely produced by phase 2 metabolism involving sulphation, acetylation or conjugation with glucuronic acid.	☐	☐
22.	Grapefruit juice induces CYP3A4 activity in the gut mucosa.	☐	☐
23.	The excretion of amphetamine is increased if the urine is strongly acid.	☐	☐
24.	Hydroxyrisperidone is an inactive metabolite.	☐	☐

25. Plasma concentration of clozapine rises significantly when fluvoxamine is added. ☐ ☐

26. The blood test for serum lithium level measurement should preferably be done 24 hours after the previous dose. ☐ ☐

27. Low plasma albumin leads to lithium toxicity. ☐ ☐

28. Increased progesterone secretion during pregnancy suppresses hepatic metabolism of drugs. ☐ ☐

29. DOPA decarboxylase converts dopamine to noradrenalin. ☐ ☐

30. D1 and D5 receptors stimulate adenylate cyclase to form cyclic – AMP as a second messenger. ☐ ☐

31. 5HT2C antagonists cause weight loss. ☐ ☐

32. 5HT2A antagonists reduce hallucinations caused by psychotomimetic drugs. ☐ ☐

33. Hallucinations may be caused by H2 antagonists (e.g. ranitidine and cimetidone). ☐ ☐

34. Labelled ligands such a raclopride and epidepride are used to measure the receptor occupancy of the antipsychotic. ☐ ☐

35. Clozapine has a low ratio of receptor-binding affinities to 5-HT2A and D2 sites. ☐ ☐

36. Nausea and insomnia are the features of cholinergic rebound following the abrupt discontinuation of anticholinergic drugs. ☐ ☐

37. Higher doses of procyclidine cause hallucinations, euphoria and dilated pupils. ☐ ☐

38. Orphenadrine has more stimulant effects than procyclidine or benzhexol. ☐ ☐

39. Hyoscine is useful in the treatment of clozapine-induced hypersalivation. ☐ ☐

40. Acamprosate is used in the treatment of alcohol detoxification. ☐ ☐

41. Lofexidine causes more hypotension than clonidine. ☐ ☐

42. Lofexidine is alpha2 adrenergic agonist used in the treatment of acute opiate withdrawal syndrome. ☐ ☐

43. Buprenorphine has both opioid agonist and antagonist actions. ☐ ☐

44. Hormone replacement therapy in women has been reported to be associated with an increased risk of developing Alzheimer's disease. ☐ ☐

45. Aspirin and dipyridamole are beneficial in the treatment of vascular dementia. ☐ ☐

46. Galantamine was originally extracted from daffodils. ☐ ☐

47. Traces of lithium are absent normally in the human body. ☐ ☐

48. A low-sodium diet increases serum lithium levels. ☐ ☐

49. PET studies have shown that the D2 receptor occupancy by clozapine is much higher than by conventional anti psychotics. ☐ ☐

50. Study of how the body handles a drug is pharmacokinetics. ☐ ☐

1. **Tubocurarine is a nicotinic receptor antagonist.**
Ans. **True.**

2. **In a dose-response curve ED50 represents the dose which elicits 50% of the maximal response and Emax represents the dose which elicits maximum response.**
Ans. **True.**

3. **IC50 represents the concentration of antagonist needed to displace the ligand from 50% of the available receptors.**
Ans. **True.**

4. **Co-administration of tryptophan and an MAOI should be avoided.**
Ans. **False.** Co-administration of tryptophan and an MAO1 is useful in the treatment of resistant depression.

5. **Mianserin causes the blockade of alpha 2 adrenoceptors and 5-HT2 receptors.**
Ans. **True.**

6. **d-serine is an NMDA receptor antagonist.**
Ans. **False.** d-serine is an NMDA receptor agonist.

7. **d-cycloserine is a partial agonist at the NMDA receptor glycine site.**
Ans. **True.**

8. **In some trials, sigma receptor antagonists have shown an antipsychotic effect.**
Ans. **True.** For example, panamesine

9. **GABA-A receptor agonists might be of some use as adjuvants in the treatment of schizophrenia.**
Ans. **True.** GABA-A receptors are inhibitory and GABA-B receptors are stimulatory on the dopamine receptors.

10. **Omega-3 fatty acids are shown to be increased in the neuronal membranes of schizophrenic patients.**
Ans. **False.** They are deficient. This is the basis of the phospholipid and membrane hypothesis.

11. **Antidepressant drugs are not associated with tolerance and craving.**
Ans. **True.**

12. **Iloperidone is a new antipsychotic with very high affinity for alpha-2 adrenoceptors.**
Ans. **True.**

13. **Methylphenidate is a controlled class B drug in the UK used in the treatment of attention deficit hyperactivity disorder.**
Ans. **True.**

14. **More than 90% of unchanged aripiprazole is renally excreted.**
Ans. **False.** Less than 1%.

15. **In the treatment of drug addiction, diamorphine can be prescribed in the UK without a special licence.**
Ans. **False:** A special licence issued by the Home Secretary is required to prescribe diamorphine (heroin), dipipanone and cocaine.

16. **Coproxamol overdosage presents with pinpoint pupils and respiratory depression.**
Ans. **True.**

17. **Neostigmine reverses the action of the depolarising muscle relaxant suxamethonium.**
Ans. **False.** It prolongs the action of suxamethonium.

18. **Anticholinesterases such as neostigmine reverse the effects of the non- depolarised muscle relaxant drugs.**

Ans. **True.**

19. **Naloxone reverses opioid-induced respiratory depression.**

Ans. **True.**

20. **Dantrolene worsens the symptoms of malignant hyperthermia.**

Ans. **False.** It is used in the treatment of malignant hyperthermia.

21. **Active metabolites are rarely produced by phase 2 metabolism involving sulphation, acetylation or conjugation with glucuronic acid.**

Ans. **True.**

22. **Grapefruit juice induces CYP3A4 activity in the gut mucosa.**

Ans. **False.** It inhibits it.

23. **The excretion of amphetamine is increased if the urine is strongly acid.**

Ans. **True.** Amphetamine is a weak base.

24. **Hydroxyrisperidone is an inactive metabolite.**

Ans. **False.** It is an active metabolite.

25. **Plasma concentration of clozapine rises significantly when fluvoxamine is added.**

Ans. **True.** Fluvoxamine inhibits CYP1A2.

26. **The blood test for serum lithium level measurement should preferably be done 24 hours after the previous dose.**

Ans. **False.** It should be done after 12 hours.

27. **Low plasma albumin leads to lithium toxicity.**

Ans. **False.** Lithium is not protein bound.

28. **Increased progesterone secretion during pregnancy suppresses hepatic metabolism of drugs.**

Ans. **True.**

29. **DOPA decarboxylase converts dopamine to noradrenalin.**

Ans. **False.** It is converted by dopamine-ß -hydroxylase.

30. **D1 and D5 receptors stimulate adenylate cyclase to form cyclic – AMP as a second messenger.**

Ans. **True.**

31. **5HT2C antagonists cause weight loss.**

Ans. **False.** They cause weight gain.

32. **5HT2A antagonists reduce hallucinations caused by psychotomimetic drugs.**

Ans. **True.**

33. **Hallucinations may be caused by H2 antagonists (e.g. ranitidine and cimetidone).**

Ans. **True.**

34. **Labelled ligands such a raclopride and epidepride are used to measure the receptor occupancy of the antipsychotic.**

Ans. **True.**

35. **Clozapine has a low ratio of receptor-binding affinities to 5-HT2A and D2 sites.**

Ans. **False.** It has a high ratio.

36. **Nausea and insomnia are the features of cholinergic rebound following the abrupt discontinuation of anticholinergic drugs.**

Ans. **True.**

37. **Higher doses of procyclidine cause hallucinations, euphoria and dilated pupils.**
Ans. **True.**

38. **Orphenadrine has more stimulant effects than procyclidine or benzhexol.**
Ans. **False.** It is less of a stimulant.

39. **Hyoscine is useful in the treatment of clozapine-induced hypersalivation.**
Ans. **True.**

40. **Acamprosate is used in the treatment of alcohol detoxification.**
Ans. **False.** It is used as an anti-craving drug for the maintenance of abstinence from alcohol.

41. **Lofexidine causes more hypotension than clonidine.**
Ans. **False:** It causes less hypotension than clonidine

42. **Lofexidine is alpha2 adrenergic agonist used in the treatment of acute opiate withdrawal syndrome.**
Ans. **True.**

43. **Buprenorphine has both opioid agonist and antagonist actions.**
Ans. **True.**

44. **Hormone replacement therapy in women has been reported to be associated with an increased risk of developing Alzheimer's disease.**
Ans. **False.** It is associated with a reduced risk.

45. **Aspirin and dipyridamole are beneficial in the treatment of vascular dementia.**
Ans. **True.**

46. **Galantamine was originally extracted from daffodils.**
Ans. **True.**

47. **Traces of lithium are absent normally in the human body.**
Ans. **False.**

48. **A low-sodium diet increases serum lithium levels.**
Ans. **True.**

49. **PET studies have shown that the D2 receptor occupancy by clozapine is much higher than by conventional anti psychotics.**
Ans. **False.** D2 receptor occupancy by clozapine is 42-60% of that of conventional anti-psychotics.

50. **Study of how the body handles a drug is pharmacokinetics.**
Ans. **True.**

Paper 3

	True	False
1. Serum lithium levels can continue to rise after treatment is stopped.	☐	☐
2. Vigabatrin causes reversible visual field defects.	☐	☐
3. Topiramate causes weight loss.	☐	☐
4. Sulpiride is excreted unchanged in the urine.	☐	☐
5. Sulpiride has activating effects at high doses.	☐	☐
6. Memantine increases the inhibition of acetylcholinesterase by donepezil.	☐	☐
7. Risperidone is more extensively hepatically metabolised than paliperidone.	☐	☐
8. In first-order elimination kinetics, the rate of elimination of a drug is not proportional to the concentration of the drug in the body.	☐	☐
9. A drug with zero-order kinetics is more likely to reach toxic levels than a drug with a first-order kinetics.	☐	☐
10. Amisulpride has an active metabolite that can be measured in the urine.	☐	☐
11. Clozapine should not be given with penicillamine.	☐	☐
12. Active metabolites with short half-lives may protect against withdrawal symptoms.	☐	☐
13. About 80 percent of the filtered lithium is reabsorbed by proximal convoluted tubule.	☐	☐
14 Tetracycline increases the risk of toxicity due to lithium.	☐	☐
15. The CYP2C19 gene is located on the short arm of chromosome 15.	☐	☐
16. In the gut most of the MAO is type B.	☐	☐
17. In the brain most of the MAO is type B.	☐	☐
18. Phase III clinical trials involve post-marketing surveillance.	☐	☐
19. Cross-tolerance can only occur between drugs with a similar mechanism of action at the cellular level.	☐	☐
20. Anandamide is an ethanolamide derivative of arachidonic acid.	☐	☐
21. Benzodiazepines with longer half-lives are more likely to cause more severe withdrawal effects.	☐	☐
22. Study of the effects of the drug on the body is 'pharmacokinetics'.	☐	☐
23. 'Median toxic dose' is the dose at which 50 percent of patients experience a toxic effect.	☐	☐
24. The ratio of the median toxic dose to the median effective dose is 'therapeutic window'.	☐	☐
25. Pindolol antagonizes the 5-HT 1A autoreceptors.	☐	☐
26. The anticholinergic activity of psychotropic drugs can cause mydriasis and cycloplegia, resulting in presbyopia.	☐	☐

27. Bethanecol is contraindicated in the treatment of adverse effects caused by blockade of muscarinic acetylcholine receptors. ☐ ☐

28. Fluvoxamine increases theophyline concentration by inhibiting CYP 1A2. ☐ ☐

29. Flavin-containing monooxygenase-3(FMO-3) is involved in the metabolism of olanzapine. ☐ ☐

30. Lithium is contraindicated in sick sinus syndrome. ☐ ☐

31. Lithium causes hyperkalemia. ☐ ☐

32. Rapid cycling, dysphoric mania and mixed affective episodes are good predictors of improvement with lithium use. ☐ ☐

33. Addition of pindolol to an SSRI can accelerate and augment the antidepressant effect. ☐ ☐

34. Compared to other antidepressants, trazodone rarely causes priapism. ☐ ☐

35. Among methods used for switching antipsychotic medications, cross-titration is less likely to cause relapse of psychosis than other methods of switching. ☐ ☐

36. Chlorpromazine reverses the antihypertensive effects of guanethidine. ☐ ☐

37. Phenylephrine can be safely given to a patient who is on MAOI. ☐ ☐

38. Aspirin can increase serum lithium levels resulting in lithium toxicity. ☐ ☐

39. Super-sensitivity due to prolonged blockade of a receptor by a drug, shifts the dose-response curve to the right. ☐ ☐

40. Anhedonic ejaculation has been reported with desipramine. ☐ ☐

41. LAAM (L-alpha acetyl methadol acetate) has shorter duration of action than methadone. ☐ ☐

42. Calcium carbamide is a more rapidly acting aldehyde dehydrogenase inhibitor than disulfiram. ☐ ☐

43. A partial agonist acts as an agonist at higher concentrations. ☐ ☐

44. Autoreceptors are postsynaptic receptors. ☐ ☐

45. Dissociation constant may be expressed as the reciprocal of the affinity constant. ☐ ☐

46. Plasma levels of zaleplon and zolpidem are decreased by rifampicin. ☐ ☐

47. Naltrexone is a shorter acting μ receptor antagonist than nalexone. ☐ ☐

48. Chronic alcohol abuse down-regulates NMDA receptors and up-regulates GABAergic receptors. ☐ ☐

49. Incidence of akathisia is more common with the use of high potency antipsychotic drugs. ☐ ☐

50. Subsensitivity due to chronic stimulation of a receptor by an agonist shifts the dose-response curve to the right. ☐ ☐

Paper 3

1. Serum lithium levels can continue to rise after treatment is stopped.
Ans. **True.** It occurs through release of intracellular lithium.

2. Vigabatrin causes reversible visual field defects.
Ans. **False.** It is irreversible.

3. Topiramate causes weight loss.
Ans. **True.**

4. Sulpiride is excreted unchanged in the urine.
Ans. **True.**

5. Sulpiride has activating effects at high doses.
Ans. **False.** It has activating effects at low doses.

6. Memantine increases the inhibition of acetylcholinesterase by donepezil.
Ans. **False.** No effect.

7. Risperidone is more extensively hepatically metabolised than paliperidone.
Ans. **True.**

8. In first-order elimination kinetics, the rate of elimination of a drug is not proportional to the concentration of the drug in the body.
Ans. **False.** The two are directly proportional.

9. A drug with zero-order kinetics is more likely to reach toxic levels than a drug with a first-order kinetics.
Ans. **True.**

10. Amisulpride has an active metabolite that can be measured in the urine.
Ans. **False:** Amisulpride is excreted unchanged in the urine.

11. Clozapine should not be given with penicillamine.
Ans. **True.** This is because they both reduce white cell count.

12. Active metabolites with short half-lives may protect against withdrawal symptoms.
Ans. **False.** Those with long half-lives do.

13. About 80 percent of the filtered lithium is reabsorbed by proximal convoluted tubule.
Ans. **True.**

14. Tetracycline increases the risk of toxicity due to lithium.
Ans. **True.**

15. The CYP2C19 gene is located on the short arm of chromosome 15.
Ans. **False.** Chromosome 10 at 10q24.1-q24.3.

16. In the gut most of the MAO is type B.
Ans. **True.**

17. In the brain most of the MAO is type B.
Ans. **True.**

18. Phase III clinical trials involve post-marketing surveillance.
Ans. **False:** Phase III trials involve full scale evaluation of treatment. Phase IV trials involve post-marketing surveillance.

19. **Cross-tolerance can only occur between drugs with a similar mechanism of action at the cellular level.**
Ans. **True.**

20. **Anandamide is an ethanolamide derivative of arachidonic acid.**
Ans. **True.**

21. **Benzodiazepines with longer half-lives are more likely to cause more severe withdrawal effects.**
Ans. **False.** Those with shorter half-lives cause more severe withdrawal symptoms.

22. **Study of the effects of the drug on the body is 'pharmacokinetics'.**
Ans. **False.** It is known as pharmacodynamics.

23. **'Median toxic dose' is the dose at which 50 percent of patients experience a toxic effect.**
Ans. **True.**

24. **The ratio of the median toxic dose to the median effective dose is 'therapeutic window'.**
Ans. **False.** It is called the therapeutic index.

25. **Pindolol antagonizes the 5-HT 1A autoreceptors.**
Ans. **True.**

26. **The anticholinergic activity of psychotropic drugs can cause mydriasis and cycloplegia, resulting in presbyopia.**
Ans. **True.**

27. **Bethanecol is contraindicated in the treatment of adverse effects caused by blockade of muscarinic acetylcholine receptors.**
Ans. **False.** It can be used as bethanecol is a cholinomimetic.

28. **Fluvoxamine increases theophyline concentration by inhibiting CYP 1A2.**
Ans. **True.**

29. **Flavin-containing monooxygenase-3(FMO-3) is involved in the metabolism of olanzapine.**
Ans. **True.**

30. **Lithium is contraindicated in sick sinus syndrome.**
Ans. **True.**

31. **Lithium causes hyperkalemia.**
Ans. **False.** It can cause a hypokalaemia-like syndrome with T-wave inversion or flattening.

32. **Rapid cycling, dysphoric mania and mixed affective episodes are good predictors of improvement with lithium use.**
Ans. **False.**

33. **Addition of pindolol to an SSRI can accelerate and augment the antidepressant effect.**
Ans. **True.**

34. **Compared to other antidepressants, trazodone rarely causes priapism.**
Ans. **False.** Trazodone causes priapism more than other antidepressants

35. **Among methods used for switching antipsychotic medications, cross-titration is less likely to cause relapse of psychosis than other methods of switching.**
Ans. **True.**

36. **Chlorpromazine reverses the antihypertensive effects of guanethidine.**
Ans. **True.**

37. **Phenylephrine can be safely given to a patient who is on MAOI.**
Ans. **False.** It can cause a hypertensive crisis.

38. Aspirin can increase serum lithium levels resulting in lithium toxicity.

Ans. False.

39. Super-sensitivity due to prolonged blockade of a receptor by a drug, shifts the dose-response curve to the right.

Ans. False. The curve is shifted to the left.

40. Anhedonic ejaculation has been reported with desipramine.

Ans. True.

41. LAAM (L-alpha acetyl methadol acetate) has shorter duration of action than methadone.

Ans. False. It has a longer duration of 3 days.

42. Calcium carbamide is a more rapidly acting aldehyde dehydrogenase inhibitor than disulfiram.

Ans. True.

43. A partial agonist acts as an agonist at higher concentrations.

Ans. False. This occurs at lower concentrations.

44. Autoreceptors are postsynaptic receptors.

Ans. False. They are presynaptic.

45. Dissociation constant may be expressed as the reciprocal of the affinity constant.

Ans. True.

46. Plasma levels of zaleplon and zolpidem are decreased by rifampicin.

Ans. True. Rifampicin induces CYP3A4.

47. Naltrexone is a shorter acting μ receptor antagonist than nalexone.

Ans. False. Naltrexone is longer acting (t ½ 1-3 days compared to naloxone's t ½ 2–4 hrs).

48. Chronic alcohol abuse down-regulates NMDA receptors and up-regulates GABAergic receptors.

Ans. False. It up-regulates NMDA receptors and down-regulates GABAergic receptors.

49. Incidence of akathisia is more common with the use of high potency antipsychotic drugs.

Ans. True.

50. Subsensitivity due to chronic stimulation of a receptor by an agonist shifts the dose-response curve to the right.

Ans. True.

Paper 4

	True	False
1. Ziprasidone causes significant weight gain.	☐	☐
2. Mirtazapine blocks 5-HT2C and H, receptors causing significant weight gain as a side effect.	☐	☐
3. SERT is a serotonin transporter protein to which both tricyclic antidepressants and SSRIs bind.	☐	☐
4. Drug treatment of people with generalized anxiety disorder who cannot tolerate SSRIs or SNRIs include pregabalin.	☐	☐
5. Controlled clinical studies do not support the use of paroxetine in the treatment of children and adolescents with major depressive disorder.	☐	☐
6. Abercanil, a new beta-carboline, has slower onset of anxiolytic action than that of the partial 5-HT1A receptor agonist buspirone.	☐	☐
7. Cholestatic jaundice due to chlorpromazine is dose-related.	☐	☐
8. Four different adenosine receptor subtypes A1, A 2A, A 2B and A3 have been identified.	☐	☐
9. Coffee and tea contain adenosine receptor antagonists.	☐	☐
10. Schizophrenia is associated with low rates of diabetes before treatment with anti psychotic drugs.	☐	☐
11. A patient currently stable on treatment with risperidone can present with symptoms of hyperprolactinaemia after the addition of paroxetine.	☐	☐
12. Renal lithium clearance is inversely proportional to its glomerular filtration.	☐	☐
13. Polymorphic A2A adenosine receptors have been implicated in panic disorders.	☐	☐
14. Lithium citrate and lithium carbonate, mg for mg, contain equal amounts of lithium.	☐	☐
15. The concentration of lithium in plasma is less than inside RBCs.	☐	☐
16. Progabide and fengabine are mixed GABA-A and GABA-B agonists with some anti-depressant properties.	☐	☐
17. 5-HT2 antagonists can improve SSRI-induced sexual dysfunction.	☐	☐
18. Zopiclone increases frequency of chloride channel opening.	☐	☐
19. O-demethylvenlafaxine is an inactive metabolite of Venlafaxine.	☐	☐
20. Pimozide and clarithromycin can be given together safely.	☐	☐
21. Lithium decreases Na /K –ATPase in patients with bipolar diorders.	☐	☐
22. Treatment with quetiapine is not associated with hyperprolactinaemia.	☐	☐
23. Clozapine has low affinity for D4 receptors.	☐	☐
24. GABA B receptors are not linked to chloride channel.	☐	☐
25. Desmethylclomipramine is an active metabolite of clomipramine.	☐	☐

	True	False

26. Lamotrigine is associated with an increased risk of switching to mania in the treatment of bipolar depression. ☐ ☐

27. Lithium has no effect on the mood of people with no history of a mood disorder. ☐ ☐

28. True steady state of a drug occurs only with a sublingual route. ☐ ☐

29. Type 2 diabetes mellitus is two-to-four times more prevalent in schizophrenia patients than in the general population. ☐ ☐

30. In the treatment of depression, 'response' to anti depressant medication can be defined by a reduction of more than 50% on a valid symptom rating scale. ☐ ☐

31. Patients with panic disorder show reduced sensitivity to yohimbine. ☐ ☐

32. Use of valproate in pregnancy is associated with cleft lip. ☐ ☐

33. Serum cortisol response to 5-hydroxy tryptophan is blunted during lithium treatment. ☐ ☐

34. Moclobemide causes significant sexual side-effects. ☐ ☐

35. Volume of distribution (Vd) of a drug is usually directly proportional to the plasma protein binding of the drug. ☐ ☐

36. Incidence densities (ID's) of events during treatment are presented as the number of reports per 1000 patient months of treatment. ☐ ☐

37. Yohimbine and clonidine should not be used together. ☐ ☐

38. Chronic lithium treatment reduces 5-HT receptor sensitivity in the hippocampus. ☐ ☐

39. Sensory neuron-specific receptors are implicated in the modulation of nociception and are insensitive to naloxone unlike opioid receptors. ☐ ☐

40. Fluvoxamine causes significant sexual dysfunction compared to other SSRIs. ☐ ☐

41. Abrupt interruption of treatment with fluoxetine is more likely to cause discontinuation reactions than with paroxetine. ☐ ☐

42. Pharmakokinetics of paroxetine, fluoxetine and fluvoxamine are non-linear. ☐ ☐

43. L-tryptophan reduces the risk of serotonin syndrome when co-administered with SSRIs. ☐ ☐

44. Fluoxetine has slower onset of antidepressant action compared with other SSRIs. ☐ ☐

45. At a given dose, plasma concentrations of sertraline and fluvoxamine are higher in elderly patients than in younger patients. ☐ ☐

46. Clomipramine, amitriptyline and imipramine are secondary amines. ☐ ☐

47. Neuroleptic malignant syndrome (NMS) is an idiosyncratic reaction to anti psychotic drugs. ☐ ☐

48. Lithium clearance decreases during pregnancy. ☐ ☐

49. Inverse benzodiazepine agonists cause severe anxiety. ☐ ☐

50. O-desmethyl venlafaxine (ODV) is an active metabolite of venlafaxine. ☐ ☐

1. Ziprasidone causes significant weight gain.

Ans. False.

2. Mirtazapine blocks 5-HT2C and H, receptors causing significant weight gain as a side effect.

Ans. True.

3. SERT is a serotonin transporter protein to which both tricyclic antidepressants and SSRIs bind.

Ans. True.

4. Drug treatment of people with generalized anxiety disorder who cannot tolerate SSRIs or SNRIs include pregabalin.

Ans. True.

5. Controlled clinical studies do not support the use of paroxetine in the treatment of children and adolescents with major depressive disorder.

Ans. True.

6. Abercanil, a new beta-carboline, has slower onset of anxiolytic action than that of the partial 5-HT1A receptor agonist buspirone.

Ans. False.

7. Cholestatic jaundice due to chlorpromazine is dose-related.

Ans. False.

8. Four different adenosine receptor subtypes A1, A 2A, A 2B and A3 have been identified.

Ans. True.

9. Coffee and tea contain adenosine receptor antagonists.

Ans. True. They contain caffeine, theophylline and theobromine which are adenosine receptor antagonists.

10. Schizophrenia is associated with low rates of diabetes before treatment with anti psychotic drugs.

Ans. False. It is associated with high rates of diabetes.

11. A patient currently stable on treatment with risperidone can present with symptoms of hyperprolactinaemia after the addition of paroxetine.

Ans. True: Paroxetine inhibits CYP 2D6 which metabolises risperidone.

12. Renal lithium clearance is inversely proportional to its glomerular filtration.

Ans. False. They are directly proportional.

13. Polymorphic A2A adenosine receptors have been implicated in panic disorders.

Ans. True.

14. Lithium citrate and lithium carbonate, mg for mg, contain equal amounts of lithium.

Ans. False.

15. The concentration of lithium in plasma is less than inside RBCs.

Ans. False.

16. Progabide and fengabine are mixed GABA-A and GABA-B agonists with some anti-depressant properties.

Ans. True.

17. 5-HT2 antagonists can improve SSRI-induced sexual dysfunction.

Ans. True.

18. Zopiclone increases frequency of chloride channel opening.

Ans. True.

19. **O-demethylvenlafaxine is an inactive metabolite of Venlafaxine.**
Ans. **False.** It is an active metabolite.

20. **Pimozide and clarithromycin can be given together safely.**
Ans. **False:** Clarithromycin inhibits CYP 3A4 which metabolises pimozide resulting in QTc interval prolongation.

21. **Lithium decreases Na /K –ATPase in patients with bipolar disorders.**
Ans. **False:** Lithium causes an increase.

22. **Treatment with quetiapine is not associated with hyperprolactinaemia.**
Ans. **True.**

23. **Clozapine has low affinity for D4 receptors.**
Ans. **False.**

24. **GABA B receptors are not linked to chloride channel.**
Ans. **True.**

25. **Desmethylclomipramine is an active metabolite of clomipramine.**
Ans. **True.**

26. **Lamotrigine is associated with an increased risk of switching to mania in the treatment of bipolar depression.**
Ans. **True.**

27. **Lithium has no effect on the mood of people with no history of a mood disorder.**
Ans. **True.**

28. **True steady state of a drug occurs only with a sublingual route.**
Ans. **False.**

29. **Type 2 diabetes mellitus is two-to-four times more prevalent in schizophrenia patients than in the general population.**
Ans. **True.**

30. **In the treatment of depression, 'response' to anti depressant medication can be defined by a reduction of more than 50% on a valid symptom rating scale.**
Ans. **True.**

31. **Patients with panic disorder show reduced sensitivity to yohimbine.**
Ans. **False.** They have an increased sensitivity.

32. **Use of valproate in pregnancy is associated with cleft lip.**
Ans. **False.** It is associated with neural tube defects.

33. **Serum cortisol response to 5-hydroxy tryptophan is blunted during lithium treatment.**
Ans. **False.** It is enhanced.

34. **Moclobemide causes significant sexual side-effects.**
Ans. **False.**

35. **Volume of distribution (Vd) of a drug is usually directly proportional to the plasma protein binding of the drug.**
Ans. **False.** They are usually inversely proportional.

36. **Incidence densities (ID's) of events during treatment are presented as the number of reports per 1000 patient months of treatment.**
Ans. **True.**

37. **Yohimbine and clonidine should not be used together.**
Ans. **True.** Both drugs have mutually cancelling effects.

38. **Chronic lithium treatment reduces 5-HT receptor sensitivity in the hippocampus.**
Ans. True.

39. **Sensory neuron-specific receptors are implicated in the modulation of nociception and are insensitive to naloxone unlike opioid receptors.**
Ans. True.

40. **Fluvoxamine causes significant sexual dysfunction compared to other SSRIs.**
Ans. False.

41. **Abrupt interruption of treatment with fluoxetine is more likely to cause discontinuation reactions than with paroxetine.**
Ans. False.

42. **Pharmakokinetics of paroxetine, fluoxetine and fluvoxamine are non-linear.**
Ans. True.

43. **L-tryptophan reduces the risk of serotonin syndrome when co-administered with SSRIs.**
Ans. False. They increase the risk.

44. **Fluoxetine has slower onset of antidepressant action compared with other SSRIs.**
Ans. True.

45. **At a given dose, plasma concentrations of sertraline and fluvoxamine are higher in elderly patients than in younger patients.**
Ans. False.

46. **Clomipramine, amitriptyline and imipramine are secondary amines.**
Ans. False. They are tertiary amines.

47. **Neuroleptic malignant syndrome (NMS) is an idiosyncratic reaction to anti psychotic drugs.**
Ans. True.

48. **Lithium clearance decreases during pregnancy.**
Ans. False. It increases.

49. **Inverse benzodiazepine agonists cause severe anxiety.**
Ans. True.

50. **O-desmethyl venlafaxine (ODV) is an active metabolite of venlafaxine.**
Ans. True.

Paper 5

	True	False
1. The incidence of EPS due to quetiapine is at placebo-level.	☐	☐
2. In the treatment of anxiety, beta-blockers act more slowly than tricyclic anti depressants.	☐	☐
3. SSRIs increase serotonergic transmission in brain stem, resulting in insomnia.	☐	☐
4. Varenicline is a selective nicotine receptor antagonist.	☐	☐
5. Nortriptyline, desipramine and protryptylin are tertiary amines.	☐	☐
6. Central serotoninergic activity can be increased by augmenting tricyclic anti depressants with lithium.	☐	☐
7. Hyperglycaemia has been less commonly associated with clozapine and olanzapine than with other atypical anti psychotic drugs.	☐	☐
8. Buspirone is effective in treating benzodiazepine withdrawal symptoms.	☐	☐
9. Sensorimotor impairment is a significant side-effect of beta-blockers used in treatment of anxiety.	☐	☐
10. Ovulation suppression by gonadotropin releasing hormone agonists (buserelin and leuprolide) is effective in the treatment of premenstrual syndrome.	☐	☐
11. Secondary amine tricyclic antidepressant drugs cause more adverse effects than tertiary amines.	☐	☐
12. Among glutamate receptors, only metabotropic glutamate receptors (MGluR) are coupled to G proteins.	☐	☐
13. Physical aspects of the medication do not influence the strength of the placebo effect.	☐	☐
14. Unionised form of acidic drugs decreases with low pH.	☐	☐
15. Amoxapine is a tetracyclic anti-depressant drug with antidopaminergic activity.	☐	☐
16. Symptoms of trazadone overdose include priapism.	☐	☐
17. Response to thyroid hormone supplementation of anti depressants is correlated with the laboratory measures of thyroid function.	☐	☐
18. Lamotrigine has been proved to be very effective in the acute treatment of mood episodes.	☐	☐
19. Tolerance may develop for the therapeutic effects of sympathomimetics in the treatment of narcolepsy.	☐	☐
20. The risk of developing Alzheimer's disease is increased by long-term treatment with non-steroidal anti-inflammatory drugs.	☐	☐
21. In treating anxiety, CCK antagonists have shown evidence of efficacy in clinical trials.	☐	☐
22. RCTs have demonstrated efficacy of clomipramine for the treatment of anxiety associated with panic disorder.	☐	☐
23. Lamotrigine has been shown to be effective in the maintenance treatment of bipolar 1 disorder as it delays the time to intervention for a mood episode (TIME).	☐	☐

24. Ziprasidone is contraindicated in patients with a known history of QT prolongation. ☐ ☐

25. Panic symptoms never worsen in the first two weeks of treatment with an SSRI. ☐ ☐

26. Atomoxetine is metabolized by the CYP2D6 pathway to 4-hydroxyatomoxetine. ☐ ☐

27. Functional neuroimaging techniques are used for the direct visualization and quantification of drug-receptor interactions. ☐ ☐

28. D_2 receptor occupancy predicts risk for hyperprolactinaemia. ☐ ☐

29. I-pyramidyl piperazine is an active metabolite of buspirone. ☐ ☐

30. Antipsychotics with higher dissociation constants induce less extra pyramidal side-effects than antipsychotics with lower dissociation constants. ☐ ☐

31. Alcohol dependence is associated with reduced GABA receptor function. ☐ ☐

32. LAAM is a partial μ agonist. ☐ ☐

33. Bupropion causes dopamine and noradrenalin reuptake inhibition. ☐ ☐

34. MAO-B metabolises 5-HT and noradrenalin. ☐ ☐

35. Trazodone decreases concentrations of digoxin and phenytoin. ☐ ☐

36. Buspirone withdrawal syndrome presents with seizures. ☐ ☐

37. Lithium induced polyuria is a significant predisposing factor to developing irreversible renal damage. ☐ ☐

38. The risk of oral clefts with diazepam is reported to be about 7in 1000 births. ☐ ☐

39. Rapid dose reduction of a conventional anti psychotic can increase the risk of developing neuroleptic malignant syndrome. ☐ ☐

40. Tetrabenazine is contraindicated in the treatment of tardive dyskinesia. ☐ ☐

41. Alcohol is an NMDA receptor agonist. ☐ ☐

42. Buspirone is more effective for acute anxiety than benzodiazepines. ☐ ☐

43. Pulmonary embolism has been reported to be associated with clozapine in the first three months of treatment. ☐ ☐

44. Cimetidine decreases blood levels of tricyclic antidepressants. ☐ ☐

45. Affinity of a drug is the ratio of the rate of dissociation (Koff) and rate of association (Kon) of the drug to the receptor. ☐ ☐

46. Zopiclone binds to the GABA β receptor complex. ☐ ☐

47. Myocarditis has been reported to be associated with clozapine in the first six to eight weeks of treatment. ☐ ☐

48. MAO-B metabolises dopamine and phenylethylamine. ☐ ☐

49. Trazodone causes sedation by adrenergic blockade. ☐ ☐

50. Chlorpromazine shows low 5 HT 2A receptor occupancy. ☐ ☐

Paper 5

1. **The incidence of EPS due to quetiapine is at placebo-level.**
Ans. True.

2. **In the treatment of anxiety, beta-blockers act more slowly than tricyclic anti depressants.**
Ans. False. They act more quickly.

3. **SSRIs increase serotonergic transmission in brain stem, resulting in insomnia.**
Ans. True.

4. **Varenicline is a selective nicotine receptor antagonist.**
Ans. False. Nicotine receptor partial agonist.

5. **Nortriptyline, desipramine and protryptylin are tertiary amines.**
Ans. False. They are secondary amines.

6. **Central serotoninergic activity can be increased by augmenting tricyclic anti depressants with lithium.**
Ans. True.

7. **Hyperglycaemia has been less commonly associated with clozapine and olanzapine than with other atypical anti psychotic drugs.**
Ans. False. It is more commonly associated with clozapine and olanzapine.

8. **Buspirone is effective in treating benzodiazepine withdrawal symptoms.**
Ans. False. It is ineffective.

9. **Sensorimotor impairment is a significant side-effect of beta-blockers used in treatment of anxiety.**
Ans. False.

10. **Ovulation suppression by gonadotropin releasing hormone agonists (buserelin and leuprolide) is effective in the treatment of premenstrual syndrome.**
Ans. True.

11. **Secondary amine tricyclic antidepressant drugs cause more adverse effects than tertiary amines.**
Ans. False. They have fewer side effects.

12. **Among glutamate receptors, only metabotropic glutamate receptors (MGluR) are coupled to G proteins.**
Ans. True.

13. **Physical aspects of the medication do not influence the strength of the placebo effect.**
Ans. False.

14. **Unionised form of acidic drugs decreases with low pH.**
Ans. Increases.

15. **Amoxapine is a tetracyclic anti-depressant drug with antidopaminergic activity.**
Ans. True.

16. **Symptoms of trazadone overdose include priapism.**
Ans. True.

17. **Response to thyroid hormone supplementation of anti depressants is correlated with the laboratory measures of thyroid function.**
Ans. False.

18. **Lamotrigine has been proved to be very effective in the acute treatment of mood episodes.**
Ans. False.

19. **Tolerance may develop for the therapeutic effects of sympathomimetics in the treatment of narcolepsy.**
Ans. True.

20. **The risk of developing Alzheimer's disease is increased by long-term treatment with non-steroidal anti-inflammatory drugs.**
Ans. False. It is decreased.

21. **In treating anxiety, CCK antagonists have shown evidence of efficacy in clinical trials.**
Ans. False.

22. **RCTs have demonstrated efficacy of clomipramine for the treatment of anxiety associated with panic disorder.**
Ans. True.

23. **Lamotrigine has been shown to be effective in the maintenance treatment of bipolar 1 disorder as it delays the time to intervention for a mood episode (TIME).**
Ans. True.

24. **Ziprasidone is contraindicated in patients with a known history of QT prolongation.**
Ans. True.

25. **Panic symptoms never worsen in the first two weeks of treatment with an SSRI.**
Ans. False.

26. **Atomoxetine is metabolized by the CYP2D6 pathway to 4-hydroxyatomoxetine.**
Ans. True.

27. **Functional neuroimaging techniques are used for the direct visualization and quantification of drug-receptor interactions.**
Ans. True.

28. **D_2 receptor occupancy predicts risk for hyperprolactinaemia.**
Ans. True.

29. **I-pyramidyl piperazine is an active metabolite of buspirone.**
Ans. True.

30. **Antipsychotics with higher dissociation constants induce less extra pyramidal side-effects than antipsychotics with lower dissociation constants.**
Ans. True.

31. **Alcohol dependence is associated with reduced GABA receptor function.**
Ans. True.

32. **LAAM is a partial μ agonist.**
Ans. False. It is a full μ agonist.

33. **Bupropion causes dopamine and noradrenalin reuptake inhibition.**
Ans. True.

34. **MAO-B metabolises 5-HT and noradrenalin.**
Ans. False. MAO-A does this.

35. **Trazodone decreases concentrations of digoxin and phenytoin.**
Ans. False. It increases this.

36. **Buspirone withdrawal syndrome presents with seizures.**
Ans. False. There is no evidence for buspirone withdrawal syndrome.

37. **Lithium induced polyuria is a significant predisposing factor to developing irreversible renal damage.**
Ans. False.

38. **The risk of oral clefts with diazepam is reported to be about 7in 1000 births.**

Ans. **True.**

39. **Rapid dose reduction of a conventional anti psychotic can increase the risk of developing neuroleptic malignant syndrome.**

Ans. **True.**

40. **Tetrabenazine is contraindicated in the treatment of tardive dyskinesia.**

Ans. **False.**

41. **Alcohol is an NMDA receptor agonist.**

Ans. **False.** It is an NMDA receptor antagonist.

42. **Buspirone is more effective for acute anxiety than benzodiazepines.**

Ans. **False.**

43. **Pulmonary embolism has been reported to be associated with clozapine in the first three months of treatment.**

Ans. **True.** In 1 in 4500 patients.

44. **Cimetidine decreases blood levels of tricyclic antidepressants.**

Ans. **False.** It increases blood levels.

45. **Affinity of a drug is the ratio of the rate of dissociation (Koff) and rate of association (Kon) of the drug to the receptor.**

Ans. **True.**

46. **Zopiclone binds to the GABA β receptor complex.**

Ans. **False.**

47. **Myocarditis has been reported to be associated with clozapine in the first six to eight weeks of treatment.**

Ans. **True.**

48. **MAO-B metabolises dopamine and phenylethylamine.**

Ans. **True.**

49. **Trazodone causes sedation by adrenergic blockade.**

Ans. **False.** Sedation occurs by histamine blockade.

50. **Chlorpromazine shows low 5 HT 2A receptor occupancy.**

Ans. **False.**

Paper 6

	True	False
1. Melatonin advances the sleep phase when it is taken in the evening in the delayed sleep phase syndrome.	☐	☐
2. Zaleplon binds to BZ1 (Omega – 1) benzodiazepine receptors.	☐	☐
3. Tryptophan reduces stages 3 and 4 NREM sleep.	☐	☐
4. REM rebound following abrupt discontinuation of benzodiazepines is associated with reduced tolerance to their effects.	☐	☐
5. Buprenorphine is a full μ agonist.	☐	☐
6. Sodium (Na+) ion-channel blockade (Type 1 antiarrhythmic action) is more common with tricyclic anti depressants.	☐	☐
7. Zotepine is a tricyclic dibenzothiepine.	☐	☐
8. Serum carbamazepine levels can be measured by gas-liquid chromatography.	☐	☐
9. Antipsychotics, typical and atypical, give rise to extrapyramidal side effects only when they exceed 78%–80% D_2 occupancy.	☐	☐
10. Clozapine is indicated in psychotic disorders occurring during the course of Parkinson's disease, in cases where standard treatment has failed.	☐	☐
11. Caffeine reduces the sleep latency.	☐	☐
12. Tardive dyskinesia is improved by antimuscarinic drugs.	☐	☐
13. Vigabatrin is associated with visual field defects.	☐	☐
14. Partial agonism at 5HT 1A receptors is associated with anxiolytic and antidepressant activity.	☐	☐
15. Caffeine can give false positive result in the dexamethasone suppression test.	☐	☐
16. Lithium is contraindicated for the treatment of self injurious behaviour.	☐	☐
17. Levoamphetamine is more potent than dextro-amphetamine.	☐	☐
18. Piracetam is indicated in adjunctive treatment of cortical myoclonus.	☐	☐
19. The ergot-derived dopamine receptor agonists have been associated with fibrotic reactions.	☐	☐
20. Doses of fosphenytoin sodium are expressed as Phenytoin Sodium Equivalents (PE).	☐	☐
21. Aripiprazole has high affinity for muscarinic receptors.	☐	☐
22. Fluvoxamine can precipitate caffeine toxicity.	☐	☐
23. Sodium valproate causes hypoammonaemia.	☐	☐
24. Rivastigmine causes more drug interactions than donepezil and galantamine.	☐	☐
25. Blood levels of an antiepileptic drug constitute a precise measure of the amount of drug entering the brain.	☐	☐

	True	False

26. If D$_2$ occupancy is high, atypicality of an antipsychotic drug is lost even in the presence of high 5-HT2 occupancy. ☐ ☐

27. Ritalinic acid is an active metabolite of methylphenidate. ☐ ☐

28. In idiopathic Parkinson's disease, antimuscarinic drugs reduce bradykinesia with no effect on rigidity. ☐ ☐

29. Bupropion is contraindicated in patients with a history of seizures. ☐ ☐

30. SSRIs cause bradycardia and do not prolong cardiac conduction. ☐ ☐

31. High 5HT2 receptor occupancy of an antipsychotic drug is essential to achieve freedom from extrapyramidal side effects. ☐ ☐

32. Plasma concentration of clozapine is decreased by caffeine intake. ☐ ☐

33. Cessation of treatment with modafinil does not cause REM sleep rebound. ☐ ☐

34. Selective melatonin receptor ML-1 agonists can worsen insomnia ☐ ☐

35. Sildenafil is ineffective in the treatment of SSRI induced sexual dysfunction. ☐ ☐

36. Cigarette smoking increases plasma olanzapine levels. ☐ ☐

37. Amphetamines reduce the duration of stages 3 and 4 NREM sleep ☐ ☐

38. Topiramate has been associated with acute myopia with secondary angle-closure glaucoma. ☐ ☐

39. Substance P is a neurokinin receptor (NK$_1$) agonist. ☐ ☐

40. Rivastigmine may worsen Parkinson's disease. ☐ ☐

41. It is essential to monitor plasma gabapentin levels to optimise gabapentin therapy in epilepsy. ☐ ☐

42. Clozapine treatment should be discontinued if the eosinophil count rises above 3000/mm^3. ☐ ☐

43. Acamprosate is indicated for the treatment of alcohol withdrawal symptoms. ☐ ☐

44. Vigabatrine, used in the treatment of West's syndrome, is a selective reversible inhibitor of GABA-transaminase. ☐ ☐

45. Buprenorphine is administered by subcutaneous route. ☐ ☐

46. Metabolites of a drug will reach steady state in the body in relation to their elimination half-lives and not those of their parent drugs. ☐ ☐

47. Tricyclic anti-depressants are indicated in the treatment of nocturnal enuresis in children. ☐ ☐

48. Donepezil has a half-life of approximately 7 hours. ☐ ☐

49. Rivastigmine has been associated with weight gain. ☐ ☐

50. Lamotrigine is indicated for the treatment of seizures associated with Lennox-Gastaut Syndrome. ☐ ☐

Paper 6

1. Melatonin advances the sleep phase when it is taken in the evening in the delayed sleep phase syndrome.
Ans. True.

2. Zaleplon binds to BZ1 (Omega – 1) benzodiazepine receptors.
Ans. True.

3. Tryptophan reduces stages 3 and 4 NREM sleep.
Ans. False. It prolongs these

4. REM rebound following abrupt discontinuation of benzodiazepines is associated with reduced tolerance to their effects.
Ans. False. It is associated with increased tolerance.

5. Buprenorphine is a full μ agonist.
Ans. False. It is a partial μ agonist.

6. Sodium (Na+) ion-channel blockade (Type 1 antiarrhythmic action) is more common with tricyclic anti depressants.
Ans. True.

7. Zotepine is a tricyclic dibenzothiepine.
Ans. True.

8. Serum carbamazepine levels can be measured by gas-liquid chromatography.
Ans. True.

9. Antipsychotics, typical and atypical, give rise to extrapyramidal side effects only when they exceed 78%–80% D_2 occupancy.
Ans. True.

10. Clozapine is indicated in psychotic disorders occurring during the course of Parkinson's disease, in cases where standard treatment has failed.
Ans. True.

11. Caffeine reduces the sleep latency.
Ans. False. It increases it.

12. Tardive dyskinesia is improved by antimuscarinic drugs.
Ans. False.

13. Vigabatrin is associated with visual field defects.
Ans. True.

14. Partial agonism at 5HT 1A receptors is associated with anxiolytic and antidepressant activity.
Ans. True.

15. Caffeine can give false positive result in the dexamethasone suppression test.
Ans. True.

16. Lithium is contraindicated for the treatment of self injurious behaviour.
Ans. False.

17. Levoamphetamine is more potent than dextro-amphetamine.
Ans. False.

18. Piracetam is indicated in adjunctive treatment of cortical myoclonus.
Ans. True.

19. **The ergot-derived dopamine receptor agonists have been associated with fibrotic reactions.**
Ans. **True.**

20. **Doses of fosphenytoin sodium are expressed as Phenytoin Sodium Equivalents (PE).**
Ans. **True.**

21. **Aripiprazole has high affinity for muscarinic receptors.**
Ans. **False.** It has no affinity for these.

22. **Fluvoxamine can precipitate caffeine toxicity.**
Ans. **True.** By inhibiting CYP1A2.

23. **Sodium valproate causes hypoammonaemia.**
Ans. **False.** It causes hyperammonaemia.

24. **Rivastigmine causes more drug interactions than donepezil and galantamine.**
Ans. **False.** Causes less drug interactions.

25. **Blood levels of an antiepileptic drug constitute a precise measure of the amount of drug entering the brain.**
Ans. **False.**

26. **If D_2 occupancy is high, atypicality of an antipsychotic drug is lost even in the presence of high 5-HT2 occupancy.**
Ans. **False.**

27. **Ritalinic acid is an active metabolite of methylphenidate.**
Ans. **False.** It is inactive.

28. **In idiopathic Parkinson's disease, antimuscarinic drugs reduce bradykinesia with no effect on rigidity.**
Ans. **False.** They reduce tremor and rigidity with little effect on bradykinesia.

29. **Bupropion is contraindicated in patients with a history of seizures.**
Ans. **True.**

30. **SSRIs cause bradycardia and do not prolong cardiac conduction.**
Ans. **True.**

31. **High 5HT2 receptor occupancy of an antipsychotic drug is essential to achieve freedom from extrapyramidal side effects.**
Ans. **False.** A low D_2 occupancy provides this

32. **Plasma concentration of clozapine is decreased by caffeine intake.**
Ans. **False.** It is increased.

33. **Cessation of treatment with modafinil does not cause REM sleep rebound.**
Ans. **True.**

34. **Selective melatonin receptor ML-1 agonists can worsen insomnia**
Ans. **False.**

35. **Sildenafil is ineffective in the treatment of SSRI induced sexual dysfunction.**
Ans. **False.**

36. **Cigarette smoking increases plasma olanzapine levels.**
Ans. **False.** Decreases.

37. **Amphetamines reduce the duration of stages 3 and 4 NREM sleep.**
Ans. **True.**

38. **Topiramate has been associated with acute myopia with secondary angle-closure glaucoma.**
Ans. **True.**

39. Substance P is a neurokinin receptor (NK$_1$) agonist.

Ans. **False.** It is a neurokinin receptor (NK$_1$) antagonist.

40. Rivastigmine may worsen Parkinson's disease.

Ans. **True.**

41. It is essential to monitor plasma gabapentin levels to optimise gabapentin therapy in epilepsy.

Ans. **False.**

42. Clozapine treatment should be discontinued if the eosinophil count rises above 3000/mm^3.

Ans. **True.**

43. Acamprosate is indicated for the treatment of alcohol withdrawal symptoms.

Ans. **False.** It is indicated for maintaining abstinence.

44. Vigabatrine, used in the treatment of West's syndrome, is a selective reversible inhibitor of GABA-transaminase.

Ans. **True.**

45. Buprenorphine is administered by subcutaneous route.

Ans. **False.** By the sublingual route.

46. Metabolites of a drug will reach steady state in the body in relation to their elimination half-lives and not those of their parent drugs.

Ans. **True.**

47. Tricyclic anti-depressants are indicated in the treatment of nocturnal enuresis in children.

Ans. **True.**

48. Donepezil has a half-life of approximately 7 hours.

Ans. **False.** It is 70 hours.

49. Rivastigmine has been associated with weight gain.

Ans. **False.** It is associated with weight loss.

50. Lamotrigine is indicated for the treatment of seizures associated with Lennox-Gastaut Syndrome.

Ans. **True.**

Paper 7

		True	False
1.	Reversible agranulocytosis is a rare adverse reaction due to mirtazapine.	☐	☐
2.	CYP3A4 and CYP2D6 are involved in the metabolism of approximately 20% of drugs.	☐	☐
3.	A high urinary ratio of debrisoquin to 4-hydroxy debrisoquin means that a person is a 'fast hydroxylator' of tricyclic anti depressants.	☐	☐
4.	The CYP1A2 gene is located on the long arm of chromosome 15 at 15q24.	☐	☐
5.	Shorter periods of untreated psychosis are associated with better and more rapid response to antipsychotic drug treatment than longer periods.	☐	☐
6.	Acamprosate prevents the harmful effects of continuous alcohol abuse.	☐	☐
7.	Rifampicin decreases the plasma concentration of buspirone.	☐	☐
8.	Lamotrigine prevents manic more than depressive relapse.	☐	☐
9.	Naturalistic studies in schizophrenia have shown that acute EPS are predictive of subsequent tardive dyskinesia.	☐	☐
10.	Lower doses of lithium may be required during pregnancy to prevent a relapse of mania.	☐	☐
11.	A formulation with poor bioavailability may not reach a plasma concentration above the minimal effective level.	☐	☐
12.	Clomipramine can cause fatal serotonin syndrome when combined with MAOIs.	☐	☐
13.	Concomitant use of valproate with lamotrigine reduces the risk of rash.	☐	☐
14.	Galantamine is contraindicated in severe renal impairment.	☐	☐
15.	Buprenorphine acts as an opioid partial agonist but not as partial antagonist.	☐	☐
16.	CYP3A4 constitutes approximately 70% of total cytochrome P450 in human intestine.	☐	☐
17.	The relationship between a drug concentration and its intensity of effect is shown as a counter clockwise hysteresis curve when there is an active metabolite.	☐	☐
18.	Amoxapine and its metabolite, 7-hydroxy-amoxapine, produce dopamine receptor blockade.	☐	☐
19.	Modes of action of agomelatin include 5HT2C antagonism.	☐	☐
20.	Intake of alcohol does not affect the pharmacokinetics of acamprosate.	☐	☐
21.	Maprotiline is a tetracyclic antidepressant.	☐	☐
22.	Flumazenil is contraindicated for the management of lorazepam overdose.	☐	☐
23.	Ocular formulation of pilocarpine has been reported to cause impairment of depth perception.	☐	☐
24.	Osmotic diuresis (mannitol or urea infusion) is contraindicated for the management of lithium toxicity.	☐	☐

25. Olanzapine and risperidone both show dose dependent occupancy of striatal D_2 receptors. ☐ ☐

26. Lyell syndrome (toxic epidermal necrolysis) is a rare side-effect of lamotrigine. ☐ ☐

27. Treatment with cholinesterase inhibitors has been associated with weight gain. ☐ ☐

28. Hypoalbuminaemia in severe liver disease is associated with increased toxicity of phenytoin. ☐ ☐

29. Diversity in body build across various ethnic groups can lead to differences in the volume of distribution of drugs that are lipophilic. ☐ ☐

30. Prevalence of tardive dystonia is estimated to be 10% in neuroleptic treated patients. ☐ ☐

31. Hepatic extraction ratio of a drug is the ratio of clearance after intravenous dosage divided by hepatic blood flow. ☐ ☐

32. Cimetidine prolongs the metabolism of moclobemide. ☐ ☐

33. Buspirone shows cross-tolerance with benzodiazepines. ☐ ☐

34. Galantamine antagonises the effect of anticholinergic medication. ☐ ☐

35. The incidence of poor metabolisers of CYP2C19 substrates is lower in Asians than in Caucasians. ☐ ☐

36. Concomitant use of tricyclic antidepressants can reduce the efficacy of lofexidine. ☐ ☐

37. Zaleplon binds selectively to the benzodiazepine type I receptor. ☐ ☐

38. Memory impairment may occur during long term use of lithium. ☐ ☐

39. Pyridostigmine is slower in action than neostigmine and has longer duration of action in the treatment of myasthenia gravis. ☐ ☐

40. Inhibition of a conditioned avoidance response is an animal test predictive of the antipsychotic potential of a drug. ☐ ☐

41. Cigarette smoking increases plasma haloperidol and clozapine levels. ☐ ☐

42. Phenobarbital inhibits the infant's sucking reflex. ☐ ☐

43. Perception and reporting of side-effects are significantly influenced by the patients' culturally determined beliefs and expectations. ☐ ☐

44. Tetrabenazine is a presynaptic monoamine depleting agent as well as postsynaptic dopamine receptor blocker. ☐ ☐

45. Re-emergence of tardive dyskinesia is common after clozapine withdrawal. ☐ ☐

46. Clozapine shows limbic selectivity over a wide dose range. ☐ ☐

47. Flibanserin is an antidepressant with 5HT1A agonist and 5HT2A antagonist actions. ☐ ☐

48. Acetazolamide decreases lithium excretion. ☐ ☐

49. The risk of drug induced teratogenecity is high from the third to the eleventh week of pregnancy. ☐ ☐

50. Pisa syndrome is a characteristic posture of tardive dystonia. ☐ ☐

Answers with explanations

1. Reversible agranulocytosis is a rare adverse reaction due to mirtazapine.
Ans. True.

2. CYP3A4 and CYP2D6 are involved in the metabolism of approximately 20% of drugs.
Ans. False. In approximately 80%.

3. A high urinary ratio of debrisoquin to 4-hydroxy debrisoquin means that a person is a 'fast hydroxylator' of tricyclic anti depressants.
Ans. False. It means they are a 'slow hydroxylator'.

4. The CYP1A2 gene is located on the long arm of chromosome 15 at 15q24.
Ans. True.

5. Shorter periods of untreated psychosis are associated with better and more rapid response to antipsychotic drug treatment than longer periods.
Ans. True.

6. Acamprosate prevents the harmful effects of continuous alcohol abuse.
Ans. False.

7. Rifampicin decreases the plasma concentration of buspirone.
Ans. True. Through the induction of CYP3A4.

8. Lamotrigine prevents manic more than depressive relapse.
Ans. False. It prevents depressive relapse.

9. Naturalistic studies in schizophrenia have shown that acute EPS are predictive of subsequent tardive dyskinesia.
Ans. True.

10. Lower doses of lithium may be required during pregnancy to prevent a relapse of mania.
Ans. False. Higher doses are required as GFR increases during pregnancy.

11. A formulation with poor bioavailability may not reach a plasma concentration above the minimal effective level.
Ans. True.

12. Clomipramine can cause fatal serotonin syndrome when combined with MAOIs.
Ans. True.

13. Concomitant use of valproate with lamotrigine reduces the risk of rash.
Ans. False. This increases the risk.

14. Galantamine is contraindicated in severe renal impairment.
Ans. True.

15. Buprenorphine acts as an opioid partial agonist but not as partial antagonist.
Ans. False. It has both agonist and antagonist actions.

16. CYP3A4 constitutes approximately 70% of total cytochrome P450 in human intestine.
Ans. True.

17. The relationship between a drug concentration and its intensity of effect is shown as a counter clockwise hysteresis curve when there is an active metabolite.
Ans. True.

18. Amoxapine and its metabolite, 7-hydroxy-amoxapine, produce dopamine receptor blockade.
Ans. True.

19. **Modes of action of agomelatin include 5HT2C antagonism.**
Ans. True.

20. **Intake of alcohol does not affect the pharmacokinetics of acamprosate.**
Ans. True.

21. **Maprotiline is a tetracyclic antidepressant.**
Ans. True.

22. **Flumazenil is contraindicated for the management of lorazepam overdose.**
Ans. False.

23. **Ocular formulation of pilocarpine has been reported to cause impairment of depth perception.**
Ans. True.

24. **Osmotic diuresis (mannitol or urea infusion) is contraindicated for the management of lithium toxicity.**
Ans. False.

25. **Olanzapine and risperidone both show dose dependent occupancy of striatal D_2 receptors.**
Ans. True.

26. **Lyell syndrome (toxic epidermal necrolysis) is a rare side-effect of lamotrigine.**
Ans. True.

27. **Treatment with cholinesterase inhibitors has been associated with weight gain.**
Ans. **False.** It is associated with weight loss.

28. **Hypoalbuminaemia in severe liver disease is associated with increased toxicity of phenytoin.**
Ans. True.

29. **Diversity in body build across various ethnic groups can lead to differences in the volume of distribution of drugs that are lipophilic.**
Ans. True.

30. **Prevalence of tardive dystonia is estimated to be 10% in neuroleptic treated patients.**
Ans. **False.** It is estimated to be 2%.

31. **Hepatic extraction ratio of a drug is the ratio of clearance after intravenous dosage divided by hepatic blood flow.**
Ans. True.

32. **Cimetidine prolongs the metabolism of moclobemide.**
Ans. True.

33. **Buspirone shows cross-tolerance with benzodiazepines.**
Ans. False.

34. **Galantamine antagonises the effect of anticholinergic medication.**
Ans. True.

35. **The incidence of poor metabolisers of CYP2C19 substrates is lower in Asians than in Caucasians.**
Ans. **False.** It is higher in Asians.

36. **Concomitant use of tricyclic antidepressants can reduce the efficacy of lofexidine.**
Ans. True.

37. **Zaleplon binds selectively to the benzodiazepine type I receptor.**
Ans. True.

38. **Memory impairment may occur during long term use of lithium.**
Ans. True.

39. **Pyridostigmine is slower in action than neostigmine and has longer duration of action in the treatment of myasthenia gravis.**

Ans. **True.**

40. **Inhibition of a conditioned avoidance response is an animal test predictive of the antipsychotic potential of a drug.**

Ans. **True.**

41. **Cigarette smoking increases plasma haloperidol and clozapine levels.**

Ans. **False.** It reduces these.

42. **Phenobarbital inhibits the infant's sucking reflex.**

Ans. **True.**

43. **Perception and reporting of side-effects are significantly influenced by the patients' culturally determined beliefs and expectations.**

Ans. **True.**

44. **Tetrabenazine is a presynaptic monoamine depleting agent as well as postsynaptic dopamine receptor blocker.**

Ans. **True.**

45. **Re-emergence of tardive dyskinesia is common after clozapine withdrawal.**

Ans. **False.**

46. **Clozapine shows limbic selectivity over a wide dose range.**

Ans. **True.**

47. **Flibanserin is an antidepressant with 5HT1A agonist and 5HT2A antagonist actions.**

Ans. **True.**

48. **Acetazolamide decreases lithium excretion.**

Ans. **False.** It increases it.

49. **The risk of drug induced teratogenecity is high from the third to the eleventh week of pregnancy.**

Ans. **True.**

50. **Pisa syndrome is a characteristic posture of tardive dystonia.**

Ans. **True.**

Paper 8

		True	False
1.	Clearance of a drug is measured in units of time divided by volume.	☐	☐
2.	Excretion of lithium is reduced by ibuprofen.	☐	☐
3.	Phenothiazines may increase risk of neutropenia when added to clozapine.	☐	☐
4.	Metabolism of haloperidol has been reported to be slower in Asians than Caucasians.	☐	☐
5.	Lipophilic drugs have low values of volume of distribution (Vd).	☐	☐
6.	Roxindole is a potent dopamine autoreceptor agonist, which also inhibits 5-HT uptake and has 5-HT$_{1A}$ agonistic actions.	☐	☐
7.	Angiotensin – II antagonists decrease plasma lithium concentration.	☐	☐
8.	Cimetidine inhibits the metabolism of valproate, carbamazepine and phenytoin.	☐	☐
9.	The incidence of poor metabolisers of CYP2D6 substrates is higher in Caucasians than in Asians.	☐	☐
10.	Zaleplon increases the sleep latency.	☐	☐
11.	2 mg of haloperidol can induce 70% striatal D$_2$ occupancy.	☐	☐
12.	Plasma clozapine levels are raised by cimetidine and lowered by phenytoin.	☐	☐
13.	Hydroxylated metabolites of the cyclic antidepressants are cleared from the body by hepatic biotransformation.	☐	☐
14.	Substance P is the neurokinin neurotransmitter that selectively binds to NK-1 receptors.	☐	☐
15.	Fluoxetine decreases plasma concentrations of carbamazepine and phenytoin.	☐	☐
16.	Activation of the D$_1$-like receptors by an agonist produces a decrease in cAMP.	☐	☐
17.	The metabolism of escitalopram is mainly mediated by CYP2C19.	☐	☐
18.	High affinity of a drug for the 5HT2C receptor increases its weight gain liability.	☐	☐
19.	Sildenafil is effective regardless of the cause of erectile dysfunction.	☐	☐
20.	Stimulant drugs are ineffective in the short-term treatment of ADHD.	☐	☐
21.	Plasma concentrations of norepinephrine are elevated during active alcohol drinking phase.	☐	☐
22.	Hydroxytetrabenazine is an inactive metabolite of tetrabenazine.	☐	☐
23.	Rivastigmine-induced nausea and vomiting are more common in males.	☐	☐
24.	Ketoconazole increases plasma concentrations of reboxetine.	☐	☐
25.	Mirtazapine is a centrally active presynaptic α2 – agonist.	☐	☐
26.	The risk of a switch to mania is greater for tricyclic antidepressants compared to SSRIs.	☐	☐

27. The risk of congenital abnormalities is dose related with valproate. ☐ ☐

28. A true drug steady state rarely occurs with a constant – rate intravenous infusion. ☐ ☐

29. D_2-like receptors are positively coupled to adenyl cyclase. ☐ ☐

30. Escitalopram may be started 14 hours after discontinuing treatment with an irreversible MAOI. ☐ ☐

31. The symptoms of serotonin syndrome include myoclonus. ☐ ☐

32. Adherence to anti psychotic medication is not effected by compliance therapy. ☐ ☐

33. Anticholinergic medication can cause euphoria. ☐ ☐

34. Methadone reaches steady state serum levels in 48 hours. ☐ ☐

35. Stimulants are more effective in treating hyperactivity than inattention. ☐ ☐

36. Atomoxetine has been shown to be effective in the treatment of adult ADHD. ☐ ☐

37. Valproate treatment in women with epilepsy is associated with risk of developing polycystic ovaries. ☐ ☐

38. Peak plasma concentrations of rivastigmine are reached after 8 hours. ☐ ☐

39. Gabapentin reduces plasma phenytoin concentrations. ☐ ☐

40. Naltrexone should be given to patients currently dependent on opioids. ☐ ☐

41. Nausea and vomiting are common side effects of galantamine. ☐ ☐

42. EC50 is the effective concentration that produces half of the Emax. ☐ ☐

43. Variants of human dopamine receptors D_2, D_3, and D_4 have been detected by 'gene cloning'. ☐ ☐

44. Both demethylated and didemethylated metabolites of escitalopram are pharmacologically active. ☐ ☐

45. Methadone is primarily metabolised by CYP2D6. ☐ ☐

46. Recognised side effects of transdermal selegiline include insomnia. ☐ ☐

47. Number needed to treat (NNT) is the reciprocal of the absolute benefit increase. ☐ ☐

48. Modafinil is pharmacologically and chemically similar to psycho -stimulants. ☐ ☐

49. Loop diuretics are safer than thiazides to use along with lithium. ☐ ☐

50. A time delay for response to a drug can occur despite decreasing plasma drug concentrations. ☐ ☐

Paper 8

1. Clearance of a drug is measured in units of time divided by volume.
Ans. **False.** It is measured by units of volume divided by time.

2. Excretion of lithium is reduced by ibuprofen.
Ans. **True.**

3. Phenothiazines may increase risk of neutropenia when added to clozapine.
Ans. **True.**

4. Metabolism of haloperidol has been reported to be slower in Asians than Caucasians.
Ans. **True.**

5. Lipophilic drugs have low values of volume of distribution (Vd).
Ans. **False.** They have high values.

6. Roxindole is a potent dopamine autoreceptor agonist, which also inhibits 5-HT uptake and has 5-HT$_{1A}$ agonistic actions.
Ans. **True.**

7. Angiotensin – II antagonists decrease plasma lithium concentration.
Ans. **False.** They decrease this by reducing lithium excretion.

8. Cimetidine inhibits the metabolism of valproate, carbamazepine and phenytoin.
Ans. **True.**

9. The incidence of poor metabolisers of CYP2D6 substrates is higher in Caucasians than in Asians.
Ans. **True.** (Caucasians 7%, Asians 1%).

10. Zaleplon increases the sleep latency.
Ans. **False.**

11. 2 mg of haloperidol can induce 70% striatal D$_2$ occupancy.
Ans. **True.**

12. Plasma clozapine levels are raised by cimetidine and lowered by phenytoin.
Ans. **True.**

13. Hydroxylated metabolites of the cyclic antidepressants are cleared from the body by hepatic biotransformation.
Ans. **False.** Cleared renally.

14. Substance P is the neurokinin neurotransmitter that selectively binds to NK-1 receptors.
Ans. **True.**

15. Fluoxetine decreases plasma concentrations of carbamazepine and phenytoin.
Ans. **False.**

16. Activation of the D$_1$-like receptors by an agonist produces a decrease in cAMP.
Ans. **False.**

17. The metabolism of escitalopram is mainly mediated by CYP2C19.
Ans. **True.**

18. High affinity of a drug for the 5HT2C receptor increases its weight gain liability.
Ans. **True.**

19. Sildenafil is effective regardless of the cause of erectile dysfunction.
Ans. **True.**

20. Stimulant drugs are ineffective in the short-term treatment of ADHD.

Ans. False.

21. Plasma concentrations of norepinephrine are elevated during active alcohol drinking phase.

Ans. True.

22. Hydroxytetrabenazine is an inactive metabolite of tetrabenazine.

Ans. False. It is an active metabolite.

23. Rivastigmine-induced nausea and vomiting are more common in males.

Ans. False. It is more common in females.

24. Ketoconazole increases plasma concentrations of reboxetine.

Ans. True. By inhibiting CYP3A4.

25. Mirtazapine is a centrally active presynaptic α2 – agonist.

Ans. False. It is an α2 – antagonist.

26. The risk of a switch to mania is greater for tricyclic antidepressants compared to SSRIs.

Ans. True.

27. The risk of congenital abnormalities is dose related with valproate.

Ans. True.

28. A true drug steady state rarely occurs with a constant – rate intravenous infusion.

Ans. False.

29. D_2-like receptors are positively coupled to adenyl cyclase.

Ans. False. They are negatively coupled.

30. Escitalopram may be started 14 hours after discontinuing treatment with an irreversible MAOI.

Ans. False. The waiting time is 14 days.

31. The symptoms of serotonin syndrome include myoclonus.

Ans. True.

32. Adherence to anti psychotic medication is not effected by compliance therapy.

Ans. False. It increases adherance.

33. Anticholinergic medication can cause euphoria.

Ans. True.

34. Methadone reaches steady state serum levels in 48 hours.

Ans. False. It takes 7 – 9 days.

35. Stimulants are more effective in treating hyperactivity than inattention.

Ans. True.

36. Atomoxetine has been shown to be effective in the treatment of adult ADHD.

Ans. True.

37. Valproate treatment in women with epilepsy is associated with risk of developing polycystic ovaries.

Ans. True.

38. Peak plasma concentrations of rivastigmine are reached after 8 hours.

Ans. False. Reached in 1 hour.

39. Gabapentin reduces plasma phenytoin concentrations.

Ans. False. There is no interaction.

40. Naltrexone should be given to patients currently dependent on opioids.

Ans. False. It may precipitate withdrawal syndrome.

41. Nausea and vomiting are common side effects of galantamine.

Ans. **True.**

42. EC50 is the effective concentration that produces half of the Emax.

Ans. **True.**

43. Variants of human dopamine receptors D_2, D_3, and D_4 have been detected by 'gene cloning'.

Ans. **True.**

44. Both demethylated and didemethylated metabolites of escitalopram are pharmacologically active.

Ans. **True.**

45. Methadone is primarily metabolised by CYP2D6.

Ans. **False.** It is metabolised by CYP3A4.

46. Recognised side effects of transdermal selegiline include insomnia.

Ans. **True.**

47. Number needed to treat (NNT) is the reciprocal of the absolute benefit increase.

Ans. **True.**

48. Modafinil is pharmacologically and chemically similar to psycho-stimulants.

Ans. **False.**

49. Loop diuretics are safer than thiazides to use along with lithium.

Ans. **True.**

50. A time delay for response to a drug can occur despite decreasing plasma drug concentrations.

Ans. **True.**

Paper 9

	True	False
1. Norfluoxetine has shorter half life than fluoxetine.	☐	☐
2. Cholinergic crisis requires more intensive anti cholinesterase treatment.	☐	☐
3. Zaleplon is metabolised by aldehyde oxidase to form 5-OXO-zaleplon which is an active metabolite.	☐	☐
4. Lorazepam may cause transient anterograde amnesia.	☐	☐
5. Bioavailability varies between branded and generic versions of the same drug.	☐	☐
6. Atypical antipsychotic drugs have a low risk: benefit ratio.	☐	☐
7. Carbamazepine reduces plasma methadone levels.	☐	☐
8. Tolerance to naltrexone develops with prolonged use.	☐	☐
9. CYP3A has the highest level of P450 in liver microsomes.	☐	☐
10. Clozapine has a higher affinity to the D4 receptor than either the D2 or D3 receptor.	☐	☐
11. Carbamazepine increases half-life of olanzapine.	☐	☐
12. The unbound(free) fraction of a drug is pharmacologically active and capable of crossing the blood-brain barrier.	☐	☐
13. Clozapine has been found effective in Meige's syndrome (blepharospasm and osomandibular dystonia).	☐	☐
14. Phenytoin increases plasma concentrations of paroxetine and mianserin.	☐	☐
15. Clomipramine hydrochloride is contraindicated in the treatment of cataplexy associated with narcolepsy.	☐	☐
16. Metronidazole causes disulfiram-like reaction with alcohol.	☐	☐
17. Tardive dyskinesia occurs less frequently in the elderly.	☐	☐
18. Recognised side-effects of zotepine include hypouricaemia.	☐	☐
19. Phase I metabolism of a drug involves conjugation.	☐	☐
20. Rifampicin increases plasma methadone levels.	☐	☐
21. Vomiting is a recognised feature of cholinergic rebound following sudden withdrawal of anticholinergic drug.	☐	☐
22. Hyponatraemia causes a fall in plasma lithium levels.	☐	☐
23. Antipsychotic induced interference with temperature regulation in NMS is a dose related side-effect.	☐	☐
24. Rates of glomerular filtration and tubular secretion are higher in neonates than adults.	☐	☐
25. No correlation has been found between therapeutic response to amitriptyline and urinary MHPG levels.	☐	☐

26. Forced swim test is an animal model used to test the potential antidepressant effect of a drug. ☐ ☐

27. Benzodiazepine withdrawal can cause depression. ☐ ☐

28. Lofepramine is a more sedating anti depressant than maprotiline. ☐ ☐

29. The risk for spina bifida associated with fetal exposure to carbamazepine is 12%. ☐ ☐

30. Bupropion causes more sexual dysfunction than SSRIs. ☐ ☐

31. Decreased drug clearance in old age is associated with increased steady-state levels unless dosing rate is accordingly reduced. ☐ ☐

32. Venlafaxine has more antimuscarinic effects than tricyclic anti depressants. ☐ ☐

33. Protein binding of drugs in children is more than in adults. ☐ ☐

34. Erythromycin causes an increase in plasma carbamazepine levels. ☐ ☐

35. Bipolar 1 patients are less likely to relapse than other bipolar groups on abrupt discontinuation of lithium. ☐ ☐

36. Elimination half-life of a drug decreases in obese individuals. ☐ ☐

37. Anterograde amnesia is a recognised side-effect of benzodiazepines. ☐ ☐

38. Aplastic anaemia is a recognised side-effect of mianserin. ☐ ☐

39. The risk for neural tube defects with fetal exposure to valproic acid is 10%. ☐ ☐

40. Glomerular filtration rate reaches adult levels by age 1 year. ☐ ☐

41. Stimulants increase aggressive behaviour in children with ADHD. ☐ ☐

42. Trazodone causes post synaptic 5HT2A receptor antagonism. ☐ ☐

43. Tianeptine enhances 5-HT uptake and has been shown to have anti depressant action. ☐ ☐

44. Older individuals have larger Vd for lipophilic drugs when compared to young individuals of the same gender. ☐ ☐

45. Dextroamphetamine has shorter duration of action than methylpheridate. ☐ ☐

46. A single episode of depression should be treated for 6 weeks after recovery. ☐ ☐

47. Depot antipsychotics do not produce severe extrapyramidal side effects at the time of administration. ☐ ☐

48. Alpha-1 acid glycoprotein (AAG) is a plasma protein responsible for drug binding. ☐ ☐

49. Priapism is a recognised side-effect of risperidone. ☐ ☐

50. Maprotiline has increased risk of convulsions at higher dosage. ☐ ☐

Paper 9

1. **Norfluoxetine has shorter half life than fluoxetine.**

Ans. **False.** It is longer (8-9 days).

2. **Cholinergic crisis requires more intensive anti cholinesterase treatment.**

Ans. **False.** It requires discontinuation of the treatment.

3. **Zaleplon is metabolised by aldehyde oxidase to form 5-OXO-zaleplon which is an active metabolite.**

Ans. **False.** All metabolites of zaleplon are inactive.

4. **Lorazepam may cause transient anterograde amnesia.**

Ans. **True.**

5. **Bioavailability varies between branded and generic versions of the same drug.**

Ans. **True.**

6. **Atypical antipsychotic drugs have a low risk: benefit ratio.**

Ans. **False.** They have a high risk: benefit ratio.

7. **Carbamazepine reduces plasma methadone levels.**

Ans. **True.**

8. **Tolerance to naltrexone develops with prolonged use.**

Ans. **False.**

9. **CYP3A has the highest level of P450 in liver microsomes.**

Ans. **True.**

10. **Clozapine has a higher affinity to the D4 receptor than either the D2 or D3 receptor.**

Ans. **True.**

11. **Carbamazepine increases half-life of olanzapine.**

Ans. **False.** It reduces the half-life.

12. **The unbound(free) fraction of a drug is pharmacologically active and capable of crossing the blood-brain barrier.**

Ans. **True.**

13. **Clozapine has been found effective in Meige's syndrome (blepharospasm and osomandibular dystonia).**

Ans. **True.**

14. **Phenytoin increases plasma concentrations of paroxetine and mianserin.**

Ans. **False.** It reduces them.

15. **Clomipramine hydrochloride is contraindicated in the treatment of cataplexy associated with narcolepsy.**

Ans. **False.** It is used as an adjunctive treatment.

16. **Metronidazole causes disulfiram-like reaction with alcohol.**

Ans. **True.**

17. **Tardive dyskinesia occurs less frequently in the elderly.**

Ans. **False.** It occurs more frequently in the elderly.

18. **Recognised side-effects of zotepine include hypouricaemia.**

Ans. **True.**

19. **Phase I metabolism of a drug involves conjugation.**

Ans. **False.** Phase II metabolism involves conjugation.

20. **Rifampicin increases plasma methadone levels.**

Ans. **False.** It reduces them.

21. **Vomiting is a recognised feature of cholinergic rebound following sudden withdrawal of anticholinergic drug.**

Ans. **True.**

22. **Hyponatraemia causes a fall in plasma lithium levels.**

Ans. **False.** Lithium levels rise.

23. **Antipsychotic induced interference with temperature regulation in NMS is a dose related side-effect.**

Ans. **False.** NMS is an idiosyncratic effect

24. **Rates of glomerular filtration and tubular secretion are higher in neonates than adults.**

Ans. **False.** They are lower in neonates.

25. **No correlation has been found between therapeutic response to amitriptyline and urinary MHPG levels.**

Ans. **True.**

26. **Forced swim test is an animal model used to test the potential antidepressant effect of a drug.**

Ans. **True.**

27. **Benzodiazepine withdrawal can cause depression.**

Ans. **True.**

28. **Lofepramine is a more sedating anti depressant than maprotiline.**

Ans. **False.** It is less sedating.

29. **The risk for spina bifida associated with fetal exposure to carbamazepine is 12%.**

Ans. **False.** It is 1%.

30. **Bupropion causes more sexual dysfunction than SSRIs.**

Ans. **False.**

31. **Decreased drug clearance in old age is associated with increased steady-state levels unless dosing rate is accordingly reduced.**

Ans. **True.**

32. **Venlafaxine has more antimuscarinic effects than tricyclic anti depressants.**

Ans. **False.** It has fewer antimuscarinic effects.

33. **Protein binding of drugs in children is more than in adults.**

Ans. **False.** Less protein binding of drugs occurs in children.

34. **Erythromycin causes an increase in plasma carbamazepine levels.**

Ans. **True.**

35. **Bipolar 1 patients are less likely to relapse than other bipolar groups on abrupt discontinuation of lithium.**

Ans. **False.** This is more likely in bipolar 1 patients.

36. **Elimination half-life of a drug decreases in obese individuals.**

Ans. **False.** It increases.

37. **Anterograde amnesia is a recognised side-effect of benzodiazepines.**

Ans. **True.**

38. **Aplastic anaemia is a recognised side-effect of mianserin.**

Ans. **True.**

39. **The risk for neural tube defects with fetal exposure to valproic acid is 10%.**

Ans. **False.** It is 1 – 2%.

40. **Glomerular filtration rate reaches adult levels by age 1 year.**
Ans. **True.**

41. **Stimulants increase aggressive behaviour in children with ADHD.**
Ans. **False.** They reduce this.

42. **Trazodone causes post synaptic 5HT2A receptor antagonism.**
Ans. **True.**

43. **Tianeptine enhances 5-HT uptake and has been shown to have anti depressant action.**
Ans. **True.**

44. **Older individuals have larger Vd for lipophilic drugs when compared to young individuals of the same gender.**
Ans. **True.**

45. **Dextroamphetamine has shorter duration of action than methylpheridate.**
Ans. **False.** It has a longer duration of action.

46. **A single episode of depression should be treated for 6 weeks after recovery.**
Ans. **False.** It should be treated for a minimum of 6 months.

47. **Depot antipsychotics do not produce severe extrapyramidal side effects at the time of administration.**
Ans. **True.** These occur a few hours after administration.

48. **Alpha-1 acid glycoprotein (AAG) is a plasma protein responsible for drug binding.**
Ans. **True.**

49. **Priapism is a recognised side-effect of risperidone.**
Ans. **True.**

50. **Maprotiline has increased risk of convulsions at higher dosage.**
Ans. **True.**

Paper 10

		True	False
1.	Symptoms of lithium toxicity in the neonate include flaccidity and poor suck reflex.	☐	☐
2.	Benzodiazepine receptors BZ_1 have low affinity for imidazopyridines.	☐	☐
3.	Venlafaxine can cause neuroleptic malignant syndrome.	☐	☐
4.	Physicochemical properties of a drug appear to be the best predictor of the amount of medication present in breast milk.	☐	☐
5.	Psychomotor retardation is a bad prognostic indicator of antidepressant response.	☐	☐
6.	Plasma levels of clozapine are higher in males than in females.	☐	☐
7.	Reboxetine can cause an increased plasma K+ concentration on prolonged administration in the elderly.	☐	☐
8.	Olanzapine causes dose dependent, transient hyperprolactinaemia.	☐	☐
9.	Topiramate has been shown to be effective in the treatment of drug-induced weight-gain.	☐	☐
10.	Untreated methadone withdrawal symptoms subside between 48–72 hours.	☐	☐
11.	α-methyltyrosine inhibits tyrosine hydroxylase activity.	☐	☐
12.	Response to lithium treatment is poorer in mixed affective episodes.	☐	☐
13.	Phase IV trials address the problems in clinical practice once a drug has been licensed.	☐	☐
14.	Hepatic drug metabolism is slower in children than in adults.	☐	☐
15.	Vitamin E has been shown to be effective in the treatment of tardive dyskinesia.	☐	☐
16.	Haloperidol induces weight gain more than zotepine.	☐	☐
17.	Cannabis can reduce serum levels of olanzapine and clozapine.	☐	☐
18.	$5\text{-}HT_3$ receptors are G-protein coupled.	☐	☐
19.	An MAOI-induced hypertensive crisis should be treated with α-adrenergic antagonists.	☐	☐
20.	Lithium is estimated to increase life expectancy by about 2 years.	☐	☐
21.	Abrupt withdrawal of anticholinergic drugs has been associated with neuroleptic malignant syndrome.	☐	☐
22.	Opioid analgesics should be used for analgesia for buprenorphine-prescribed patients.	☐	☐
23.	Quetiapine has been associated with raised plasma lipids.	☐	☐
24.	Carbidopa cannot prevent the conversion of L-Dopa to dopamine in brain.	☐	☐
25.	Glutamate in the glia cell is converted into glutamine by glutamine hydroxylase.	☐	☐
26.	Fluvoxamine may raise olanzapine levels.	☐	☐

	True	False

27. Manic relapse rates are higher than depressive relapse rates in patients taking lithium. ☐ ☐

28. QTc prolongation is least prominent at trough drug plasma levels. ☐ ☐

29. Higher serum lithium levels are required for the prophylactic treatment of bipolar disorder than for acute mania. ☐ ☐

30. Zotepine is associated with a high incidence of seizures. ☐ ☐

31. α-methylparatyrosine induces the hydroxylation of tyrosine which is the rate-limiting step in dopamine synthesis. ☐ ☐

32. Valproate induced congenital abnormalities are dose-related. ☐ ☐

33. Antagonists cause shift to the left in the dose-response curve for the agonist. ☐ ☐

34. Antipsychotic drugs can be started at a higher dose if the patient is presenting with severe psychosis following the recovery of neuroleptic malignant syndrome. ☐ ☐

35. A sodium-dependent plasma membrane transporter protein causes a reduction of synaptic dopamine concentration by an active reuptake process. ☐ ☐

36. 9-OH risperidone is an inactive metabolite formed by hydroxylation of risperidone. ☐ ☐

37. The evidence supporting the use of antidepressants in the long-term prophylaxis of bipolar patients is stronger than in unipolar patients. ☐ ☐

38. Flumazenil reverses the effects of lorazepam. ☐ ☐

39. $5HT_1$ receptors are inhibitory. ☐ ☐

40. Lithium discontinuation leads to a recurrence of the affective disorder in 3 months for 50% of patients. ☐ ☐

41. NICE guidance on atypical antipsychotics says that the choice of antipsychotic should be made jointly by the prescriber and the patient and/or carer. ☐ ☐

42. Glutamine is converted into glutamate by an enzyme in ribosomes. ☐ ☐

43. Ziprasidone does not cause significant QTc prolongation. ☐ ☐

44. Buprenorphine withdrawal syndrome is milder than methadone withdrawal syndrome. ☐ ☐

45. The CYP2C9 gene is located on the long arm of chromosome 22. ☐ ☐

46. Aripiprazole is a potent antagonist at $5HT_{2A}$ receptors . ☐ ☐

47. Therapeutic plasma concentrations of a drug can be achieved quicker with large initial doses. ☐ ☐

48. Zuclopenthixol acetate can be administered as a test dose for zuclopenthixol decanoate depot injection. ☐ ☐

49. Flavin adenine dinucleotide is a cofactor for both MAO-A and MAO-B enzymes. ☐ ☐

50. Metencephalin inhibits GABA inhibition of dopamine in the ventro tegmental area. ☐ ☐

Paper 10

1. **Symptoms of lithium toxicity in the neonate include flaccidity and poor suck reflex.**
Ans. **True.**

2. **Benzodiazepine receptors BZ_1 have low affinity for imidazopyridines.**
Ans. **False.** They have a high affinity.

3. **Venlafaxine can cause neuroleptic malignant syndrome.**
Ans. **True.**

4. **Physicochemical properties of a drug appear to be the best predictor of the amount of medication present in breast milk.**
Ans. **True.**

5. **Psychomotor retardation is a bad prognostic indicator of antidepressant response.**
Ans. **False.** It is a good indicator.

6. **Plasma levels of clozapine are higher in males than in females.**
Ans. **False.** They are lower in males.

7. **Reboxetine can cause an increased plasma K+ concentration on prolonged administration in the elderly.**
Ans. **False.** It lowers plasma K+ concentration.

8. **Olanzapine causes dose dependent, transient hyperprolactinaemia.**
Ans. **True.**

9. **Topiramate has been shown to be effective in the treatment of drug-induced weight-gain.**
Ans. **True.**

10. **Untreated methadone withdrawal symptoms subside between 48–72 hours.**
Ans. **False.** They take 10-12 days to subside.

11. **α-methyltyrosine inhibits tyrosine hydroxylase activity.**
Ans. **True.**

12. **Response to lithium treatment is poorer in mixed affective episodes.**
Ans. **True.**

13. **Phase IV trials address the problems in clinical practice once a drug has been licensed.**
Ans. **True.**

14. **Hepatic drug metabolism is slower in children than in adults.**
Ans. **False.** It is faster in children.

15. **Vitamin E has been shown to be effective in the treatment of tardive dyskinesia.**
Ans. **True.**

16. **Haloperidol induces weight gain more than zotepine.**
Ans. **False.**

17. **Cannabis can reduce serum levels of olanzapine and clozapine.**
Ans. **True.** Cannabis induces CYP1A2.

18. **5-HT_3 receptors are G-protein coupled.**
Ans. **False.** Ion channel-linked.

19. **An MAOI-induced hypertensive crisis should be treated with α-adrenergic antagonists.**
Ans. **True.**

20. Lithium is estimated to increase life expectancy by about 2 years.
Ans. **False.** Life expectancy is increased by 7 years.

21. Abrupt withdrawal of anticholinergic drugs has been associated with neuroleptic malignant syndrome.
Ans. **True.**

22. Opioid analgesics should be used for analgesia for buprenorphine-prescribed patients.
Ans. **False.** They should use non-opioid analgesics.

23. Quetiapine has been associated with raised plasma lipids.
Ans. **True.**

24. Carbidopa cannot prevent the conversion of L-Dopa to dopamine in brain.
Ans. **True.** Carbidopa does not cross the blood-brain-barrier.

25. Glutamate in the glia cell is converted into glutamine by glutamine hydroxylase.
Ans. **False.** It is converted by glutamine synthetase.

26. Fluvoxamine may raise olanzapine levels.
Ans. **True.** By the inhibition of CYP1A2.

27. Manic relapse rates are higher than depressive relapse rates in patients taking lithium.
Ans. **False.** Manic relapses are less common.

28. QTc prolongation is least prominent at trough drug plasma levels.
Ans. **True.**

29. Higher serum lithium levels are required for the prophylactic treatment of bipolar disorder than for acute mania.
Ans. **False.** Lower levels are needed.

30. Zotepine is associated with a high incidence of seizures.
Ans. **True.**

31. α-methylparatyrosine induces the hydroxylation of tyrosine which is the rate-limiting step in dopamine synthesis.
Ans. **True.**

32. Valproate induced congenital abnormalities are dose-related.
Ans. **True.**

33. Antagonists cause shift to the left in the dose-response curve for the agonist.
Ans. **False.** They cause a shift to the right.

34. Antipsychotic drugs can be started at a higher dose if the patient is presenting with severe psychosis following the recovery of neuroleptic malignant syndrome.
Ans. **False.** They should be started at very low dose.

35. A sodium-dependent plasma membrane transporter protein causes a reduction of synaptic dopamine concentration by an active reuptake process.
Ans. **True.**

36. 9-OH risperidone is an inactive metabolite formed by hydroxylation of risperidone.
Ans. **False.** It is an active metabolite.

37. The evidence supporting the use of antidepressants in the long-term prophylaxis of bipolar patients is stronger than in unipolar patients.
Ans. **False.** It is stronger for unipolar patients.

38. Flumazenil reverses the effects of lorazepam.
Ans. **True.**

39. **5HT$_1$ receptors are inhibitory.**
Ans. True.

40. **Lithium discontinuation leads to a recurrence of the affective disorder in 3 months for 50% of patients.**
Ans. True.

41. **NICE guidance on atypical antipsychotics says that the choice of antipsychotic should be made jointly by the prescriber and the patient and/or carer.**
Ans. True.

42. **Glutamine is converted into glutamate by an enzyme in ribosomes.**
Ans. **True.** By inducing CYP1A2.

43. **Ziprasidone does not cause significant QTc prolongation.**
Ans. False.

44. **Buprenorphine withdrawal syndrome is milder than methadone withdrawal syndrome.**
Ans. True.

45. **The CYP2C9 gene is located on the long arm of chromosome 22.**
Ans. **False.** Chromosome 10 at 10q24.

46. **Aripiprazole is a potent antagonist at 5HT$_{2A}$ receptors.**
Ans. True.

47. **Therapeutic plasma concentrations of a drug can be achieved quicker with large initial doses.**
Ans. True.

48. **Zuclopenthixol acetate can be administered as a test dose for zuclopenthixol decanoate depot injection.**
Ans. False.

49. **Flavin adenine dinucleotide is a cofactor for both MAO-A and MAO-B enzymes.**
Ans. True.

50. **Metencephalin inhibits GABA inhibition of dopamine in the ventro tegmental area.**
Ans. True.

Paper 11

	True	False
1. Response to lithium treatment is poor in about 10% of bipolar patients.	☐	☐
2. For patients unresponsive to two different antipsychotics (one an atypical) clozapine should be considered.	☐	☐
3. Norfluoxetine is an active metabolite of fluoxetine.	☐	☐
4. Non competitive antagonists cannot be displaced by agonists.	☐	☐
5. Disinhibition reactions due to benzodiazepines are less common in those with pre-existing brain damage.	☐	☐
6. Clozapine induced diabetes mostly occurs in the first 6 months of treatment.	☐	☐
7. 5HT2C receptors are associated with food intake and anxiety.	☐	☐
8. Antipsyhchotic induced extrapyramidal side effects are more common among smokers than non-smokers.	☐	☐
9. Treatment non adherence is associated with poor doctor-patient communication.	☐	☐
10. The genes for both MAO-A and MAO-B are located on the long arm of the human X chromosome.	☐	☐
11. Cholecystokinin can inhibit panic attacks.	☐	☐
12. A manic episode followed by a depressive episode is a predictor of good response to lithium treatment.	☐	☐
13. Glutamate's actions are stopped by enzymatic breakdown.	☐	☐
14. Carbamazepine is both a substrate and an inducer of CYP 3A4.	☐	☐
15. Norrie's disease is an inherited disorder characterised by deletion of the genes for both MAO-A and MAO-B.	☐	☐
16. Tranylcypromine has mild stimulant effect.	☐	☐
17. Normal QTc limits for men are between 480 ms and 500 ms.	☐	☐
18. Phenytoin prevents alcohol withdrawal seizures.	☐	☐
19. GABA is a slow acting inhibitory neurotransmitter.	☐	☐
20. Muscarinic receptors are involved in fast synaptic transmission.	☐	☐
21. No correlation is seen between a child's serum methylphenidate levels and treatment response.	☐	☐
22. Haloperidol has histaminic and muscarinic binding activities.	☐	☐
23. Nicotine withdrawal symptoms include depressed mood.	☐	☐
24. Extrapyramidal side effects with conventional antipsychotics are more common in patients with bipolar disorders.	☐	☐
25. The risk of diabetes with clozapine is less than with conventional antipsychotic drugs.	☐	☐

26. Drugs that inhibit choline acetyl transferase (CAT) are used in the treatment of Alzheimer's disease. ☐   ☐

27. Previous history of good response to lithium treatment is a predictor of good response to lithium for the current episode. ☐   ☐

28. Amines that are present inside stored vesicles can be metabolized by MAO. ☐   ☐

29. The blood-brain barrier is absent in the anterior perforated substance and the area postrema in the floor of the fourth ventricle. ☐   ☐

30. Phenothiazines antagonise the central effects of amphetamine. ☐   ☐

31. Buprenorphine is a partial opioid agonist with high affinity at μ-opioid receptors. ☐   ☐

32. Nicotinic receptors are ion channel-linked receptors. ☐   ☐

33. Desmopressin is taken sublingually in the treatment of nocturnal enuresis. ☐   ☐

34. Atypical antipsychotics causing frequent extra pyramidal symptoms include perospirone. ☐   ☐

35. Serotonin inhibits prolactin secretion in the tubero infundibular pathway. ☐   ☐

36. Centrally-acting anticholinergics augment the antiparkinsonian effects of dopamine agonists. ☐   ☐

37. Tropolone is an inhibitor of catechol-o-methyl transferase. ☐   ☐

38. The kainate receptor is a type of glutamate receptors which is linked to ion channels. ☐   ☐

39. Doses of a drug given at longer intervals than half-life of the drug lead to less fluctuations in plasma concentration. ☐   ☐

40. Parkinson's disease occurs more frequently in smokers than in non-smokers. ☐   ☐

41. An increased number of previous manic episodes is associated with a poor response to lithium treatment. ☐   ☐

42. Peripheral neuropathy is a rare side effect of MAOIs. ☐   ☐

43. Alkalinizing the urine delays amphetamine excretion and raises plasma amphetamine levels. ☐   ☐

44. Lithium can cause mild impairment of attention and memory. ☐   ☐

45. Zuclopenthixol acetate is the drug of choice in rapid transquilisation (RT). ☐   ☐

46. One of the metabolites of moclobemide inhibits MAO-B. ☐   ☐

47. Centrally acting anticholinergics can increase the risk of tardive dyskinesia in patients treated with neuroleptics. ☐   ☐

48. Healthy young female volunteers are generally used in Phase 1 drug trials. ☐   ☐

49. The response rate to nortriptyline increases at levels above 150 ng/ml. ☐   ☐

50. Glutamate antagonists can show neuro-protective properties by blocking excitotoxic neurotransmission. ☐   ☐

Paper 11

1. **Response to lithium treatment is poor in about 10% of bipolar patients.**
Ans. **False.** It is poor in about 40%.

2. **For patients unresponsive to two different antipsychotics (one an atypical) clozapine should be considered.**
Ans. **True.**

3. **Norfluoxetine is an active metabolite of fluoxetine.**
Ans. **True.**

4. **Non competitive antagonists cannot be displaced by agonists.**
Ans. **True.**

5. **Disinhibition reactions due to benzodiazepines are less common in those with pre-existing brain damage.**
Ans. **False.** They are more common in these individuals.

6. **Clozapine induced diabetes mostly occurs in the first 6 months of treatment.**
Ans. **True.**

7. **$5HT_{2C}$ receptors are associated with food intake and anxiety.**
Ans. **True.**

8. **Antipsyhchotic induced extrapyramidal side effects are more common among smokers than non-smokers.**
Ans. **False.** They are less common among smokers.

9. **Treatment non adherence is associated with poor doctor-patient communication.**
Ans. **True.**

10. **The genes for both MAO-A and MAO-B are located on the long arm of the human X chromosome.**
Ans. **False.** They are on the short arm.

11. **Cholecystokinin can inhibit panic attacks.**
Ans. **False.** It can induce panic attacks.

12. **A manic episode followed by a depressive episode is a predictor of good response to lithium treatment.**
Ans. **True.**

13. **Glutamate's actions are stopped by enzymatic breakdown.**
Ans. **False.** They are stopped by transport pumps.

14. **Carbamazepine is both a substrate and an inducer of CYP 3A4.**
Ans. **True.**

15. **Norrie's disease is an inherited disorder characterised by deletion of the genes for both MAO-A and MAO-B.**
Ans. **True.** It presents with severe learning disability and blindness.

16. **Tranylcypromine has mild stimulant effect.**
Ans. **True.**

17. **Normal QTc limits for men are between 480 ms and 500 ms.**
Ans. **False.** Less than 440ms in men.

18. **Phenytoin prevents alcohol withdrawal seizures.**
Ans. **False.**

19. **GABA is a slow acting inhibitory neurotransmitter.**
Ans. **False.** It is fast acting.

20. **Muscarinic receptors are involved in fast synaptic transmission.**
Ans. **False.** Slow synaptic transmission (they are G-protein coupled).

21. **No correlation is seen between a child's serum methylphenidate levels and treatment response.**
Ans. **True.**

22. **Haloperidol has histaminic and muscarinic binding activities.**
Ans. **False.**

23. **Nicotine withdrawal symptoms include depressed mood.**
Ans. **True.**

24. **Extrapyramidal side effects with conventional antipsychotics are more common in patients with bipolar disorders.**
Ans. **True.**

25. **The risk of diabetes with clozapine is less than with conventional antipsychotic drugs.**
Ans. **False.** The risk in increased.

26. **Drugs that inhibit choline acetyl transferase (CAT) are used in the treatment of Alzheimer's disease.**
Ans. **False.** Acetylcholine esterase inhibitors are used to treat Alzheimer's.

27. **Previous history of good response to lithium treatment is a predictor of good response to lithium for the current episode.**
Ans. **True.**

28. **Amines that are present inside stored vesicles can be metabolized by MAO.**
Ans. **False.** MAO metabolizes only amines that are present in the cytoplasm.

29. **The blood-brain barrier is absent in the anterior perforated substance and the area postrema in the floor of the fourth ventricle.**
Ans. **True.**

30. **Phenothiazines antagonise the central effects of amphetamine.**
Ans. **True.**

31. **Buprenorphine is a partial opioid agonist with high affinity at μ-opioid receptors.**
Ans. **True.**

32. **Nicotinic receptors are ion channel-linked receptors.**
Ans. **True.**

33. **Desmopressin is taken sublingually in the treatment of nocturnal enuresis.**
Ans. **False.** It is taken nasally.

34. **Atypical antipsychotics causing frequent extra pyramidal symptoms include perospirone.**
Ans. **True.**

35. **Serotonin inhibits prolactin secretion in the tubero infundibular pathway.**
Ans. **False.** Serotonin stimulates this.

36. **Centrally-acting anticholinergics augment the antiparkinsonian effects of dopamine agonists.**
Ans. **True.**

37. **Tropolone is an inhibitor of catechol-o-methyl transferase.**
Ans. **True.**

38. **The kainate receptor is a type of glutamate receptors which is linked to ion channels.**
Ans. **True.**

39. **Doses of a drug given at longer intervals than half-life of the drug lead to less fluctuations in plasma concentration.**

Ans. **False.** This leads to more fluctuations.

40. **Parkinson's disease occurs more frequently in smokers than in non-smokers.**

Ans. **False.** It occurs less frequently.

41. **An increased number of previous manic episodes is associated with a poor response to lithium treatment.**

Ans. **True.**

42. **Peripheral neuropathy is a rare side effect of MAOIs.**

Ans. **True.**

43. **Alkalinizing the urine delays amphetamine excretion and raises plasma amphetamine levels.**

Ans. **True.**

44. **Lithium can cause mild impairment of attention and memory.**

Ans. **True.**

45. **Zuclopenthixol acetate is the drug of choice in rapid transquilisation (RT).**

Ans. **False.**

46. **One of the metabolites of moclobemide inhibits MAO-B.**

Ans. **True.**

47. **Centrally acting anticholinergics can increase the risk of tardive dyskinesia in patients treated with neuroleptics.**

Ans. **True.**

48. **Healthy young female volunteers are generally used in Phase 1 drug trials.**

Ans. **False.** They generally use males.

49. **The response rate to nortriptyline increases at levels above 150 ng/ml.**

Ans. **False.** It decreases at these levels.

50. **Glutamate antagonists can show neuro-protective properties by blocking excitotoxic neurotransmission.**

Ans. **True.**

Paper 12

		True	False
1.	MAOIs are contraindicated in patients with pheochromocytoma.	☐	☐
2.	Clozapine's affinity for D_4 receptors is much lower than its affinity for D_2 receptors.	☐	☐
3.	D_1 and D_5 receptors have a low binding affinity to [³H] spiperone.	☐	☐
4.	Benzodiazepines can be used maximum 4 weeks to treat severe and disabling anxiety.	☐	☐
5.	Bioavailability of many drugs is higher in children than in adults.	☐	☐
6.	Olanzapine and clozapine may increase the risk of gestational diabetes.	☐	☐
7.	Lithium can be useful in reversal of neutropenia.	☐	☐
8.	Steady-state level of a drug is achieved after 2 drug half-lives.	☐	☐
9.	Magnetic resonance spectroscopy has shown that it takes 6 months of regular treatment with fluoxetine to reach maximum concentrations in the brain.	☐	☐
10.	The fenfluramine-induced prolactin response is blocked by clozapine.	☐	☐
11.	The normal starting dose of an SSRI for the treatment of GAD is at half the normal starting dose for the treatment of depression.	☐	☐
12.	Antipsychotic discontinuation symptoms are not reported in the neonate.	☐	☐
13.	Suicide rate increases following discontinuation of lithium treatment.	☐	☐
14.	Cimetidine increases the clearance of moclobemide.	☐	☐
15.	Licence to market a drug is obtained before phase III drug trials.	☐	☐
16.	A low urinary norepinephrine to epinephrine ratio is seen in some depressed patients.	☐	☐
17.	The lower the equilibrium dissociation constant (Ki) of a drug, the higher its binding affinity to the receptors.	☐	☐
18.	The early development of drug induced extrapyramidal side effects is a risk factor for the development of tardive dyskinesia.	☐	☐
19.	Many drugs cross the blood-brain barrier more readily in adults than in children.	☐	☐
20.	Placebo response rates are higher among more chronically ill patients than in acutely ill patients.	☐	☐
21.	Elevated levels of urinary serotonin metabolite 5-hydroxyindoleacetic acid (5-HIAA) are noted in patients with carcinoid tumours.	☐	☐
22.	Doxepin is a highly potent H_1 histamine receptor antagonist.	☐	☐
23.	Zolpidem is a benzodiazepine partial agonist with high selectivity for GABA-B receptors containing α subunits.	☐	☐
24.	DNA microarray technology is used to identify the disease specific markers.	☐	☐

	True	False

25. Reduction in prolactin levels is seen after switching from oral risperidone to long acting injection. ☐ ☐

26. Inhibition of conditioned responses and apomorphine-induced hyperactivity in the animal model is related to antipsychotic efficacy. ☐ ☐

27. D_2 receptors are negatively coupled to adenylate cyclase and show high binding affinity to [^{3}H] spiperone. ☐ ☐

28. Clozapine may increase the risk of neonatal seizures. ☐ ☐

29. L-Alanine is an antagonist at the inhibitory glycine receptor. ☐ ☐

30. In development of a drug, purity of the compound is tested before the 'R-number' is given to the compound. ☐ ☐

31. Plasma leptin levels increase more after olanzapine treatment than after risperidone treatment. ☐ ☐

32. Administration of IV injection of sodium lactate to patients with panic disorder improves the panic attacks. ☐ ☐

33. Antagonism of apomorphine induced abnormal behaviour in rats by a drug is considered to reflect central D_2 –antagonism. ☐ ☐

34. Vigabatrin is a selective GABA – transaminase inhibitor with anticonvulsant action. ☐ ☐

35. Peak plasma level fluctuations with long acting risperidone injection are higher than with oral formulation. ☐ ☐

36. Genetic polymorphism of 5HT2C receptor and leptin promoter have been shown to predict the severity of antipsychotic induced weight gain. ☐ ☐

37. Lithium potentiates the effects of non-depolarising neuromuscular blockers. ☐ ☐

38. Use of tricyclic antidepressants in the third trimester has been associated with neonatal withdrawal effects. ☐ ☐

39. Picrotoxin is a $GABA_A$ receptor agonist. ☐ ☐

40. A single episode of depression should be treated for 6 months after recovery. ☐ ☐

41. Physostigmine improves anticholinergic toxicity by increasing the amount of acetylcholine available for synaptic transmission. ☐ ☐

42. Propranolol can impair serum glucose regulation. ☐ ☐

43. Tardive dyskinesia tends to deteriorate in time. ☐ ☐

44. Alcohol increases excitatory neurotransmission at glutamate NMDA receptors. ☐ ☐

45. Risperidone decreases deep, slow-wave sleep. ☐ ☐

46. Gabapentin has anxiolytic and antinociceptive actions. ☐ ☐

47. Cryopreserved human hepatocytes can be used as an in vitro tool to study the induction of cytochrome P450 enzymes. ☐ ☐

48. Olanzapine is less likely to cause diabetes than conventional antipsychotics. ☐ ☐

49. **More-hydrophilic β-adrenergic antagonists are more effective than the more-lipophilic ones for the treatment of akathisia.** ☐ ☐

50. **Atomoxetine should not be prescribed in combination with MAOIs.** ☐ ☐

Paper 12

1. **MAOIs are contraindicated in patients with pheochromocytoma.**
Ans. **True.**

2. **Clozapine's affinity for D_4 receptors is much lower than its affinity for D_2 receptors.**
Ans. **False.** It is higher.

3. **D_1 and D_5 receptors have a low binding affinity to [^{3}H] spiperone.**
Ans. **True.**

4. **Benzodiazepines can be used maximum 4 weeks to treat severe and disabling anxiety.**
Ans. **True.**

5. **Bioavailability of many drugs is higher in children than in adults.**
Ans. **False.** It is lower as children have a faster metabolism and the drug is distributed in a larger extracellular space.

6. **Olanzapine and clozapine may increase the risk of gestational diabetes.**
Ans. **True.**

7. **Lithium can be useful in reversal of neutropenia.**
Ans. **True.**

8. **Steady-state level of a drug is achieved after 2 drug half-lives.**
Ans. **False.** It occurs after 5 drug half-lives.

9. **Magnetic resonance spectroscopy has shown that it takes 6 months of regular treatment with fluoxetine to reach maximum concentrations in the brain.**
Ans. **True.**

10. **The fenfluramine-induced prolactin response is blocked by clozapine.**
Ans. **True.**

11. **The normal starting dose of an SSRI for the treatment of GAD is at half the normal starting dose for the treatment of depression.**
Ans. **True.**

12. **Antipsychotic discontinuation symptoms are not reported in the neonate.**
Ans. **False.**

13. **Suicide rate increases following discontinuation of lithium treatment.**
Ans. **True.**

14. **Cimetidine increases the clearance of moclobemide.**
Ans. **False.** It reduces it.'

15. **Licence to market a drug is obtained before phase III drug trials.**
Ans. **False.** This happens after phase III trials.

16. **A low urinary norepinephrine to epinephrine ratio is seen in some depressed patients.**
Ans. **True.**

17. **The lower the equilibrium dissociation constant (Ki) of a drug, the higher its binding affinity to the receptors.**
Ans. **True.**

18. **The early development of drug induced extrapyramidal side effects is a risk factor for the development of tardive dyskinesia.**
Ans. **True.**

19. Many drugs cross the blood-brain barrier more readily in adults than in children.
Ans. **False.** More readily in children.

20. Placebo response rates are higher among more chronically ill patients than in acutely ill patients.
Ans. **False.** They are lower.

21. Elevated levels of urinary serotonin metabolite 5-hydroxyindoleacetic acid (5-HIAA) are noted in patients with carcinoid tumours.
Ans. **True.**

22. Doxepin is a highly potent H_1 histamine receptor antagonist.
Ans. **True.**

23. Zolpidem is a benzodiazepine partial agonist with high selectivity for GABA-B receptors containing α subunits.
Ans. **False.** $GABA_A$ receptors.

24. DNA microarray technology is used to identify the disease specific markers.
Ans. **True.**

25. Reduction in prolactin levels is seen after switching from oral risperidone to long acting injection.
Ans. **True.**

26. Inhibition of conditioned responses and apomorphine-induced hyperactivity in the animal model is related to antipsychotic efficacy.
Ans. **True.**

27. D_2 receptors are negatively coupled to adenylate cyclase and show high binding affinity to $[^3H]$ spiperone.
Ans. **True.**

28. Clozapine may increase the risk of neonatal seizures.
Ans. **True.**

29. L-Alanine is an antagonist at the inhibitory glycine receptor.
Ans. **False.** Agonist.

30. In development of a drug, purity of the compound is tested before the 'R-number' is given to the compound.
Ans. **True.**

31. Plasma leptin levels increase more after olanzapine treatment than after risperidone treatment.
Ans. **True.**

32. Administration of IV injection of sodium lactate to patients with panic disorder improves the panic attacks.
Ans. **False.** It precipitates panic attacks.

33. Antagonism of apomorphine induced abnormal behaviour in rats by a drug is considered to reflect central D_2 –antagonism.
Ans. **True.**

34. Vigabatrin is a selective GABA – transaminase inhibitor with anticonvulsant action.
Ans. **True.**

35. Peak plasma level fluctuations with long acting risperidone injection are higher than with oral formulation.
Ans. **False.** They are lower.

36. Genetic polymorphism of 5HT2C receptor and leptin promoter have been shown to predict the severity of antipsychotic induced weight gain.
Ans. **True.**

37. **Lithium potentiates the effects of non-depolarising neuromuscular blockers.**

Ans. **True.**

38. **Use of tricyclic antidepressants in the third trimester has been associated with neonatal withdrawal effects.**

Ans. **True.** This include irritability and agitation.

39. **Picrotoxin is a GABA$_A$ receptor agonist.**

Ans. **False.** It is an antagonist.

40. **A single episode of depression should be treated for 6 months after recovery.**

Ans. **True.**

41. **Physostigmine improves anticholinergic toxicity by increasing the amount of acetylcholine available for synaptic transmission.**

Ans. **True.**

42. **Propranolol can impair serum glucose regulation.**

Ans. **True.**

43. **Tardive dyskinesia tends to deteriorate in time.**

Ans. **False.** It tends to improve.

44. **Alcohol increases excitatory neurotransmission at glutamate NMDA receptors.**

Ans. **False.** Reduces.

45. **Risperidone decreases deep, slow-wave sleep.**

Ans. **False.** Increases.

46. **Gabapentin has anxiolytic and antinociceptive actions.**

Ans. **True.**

47. **Cryopreserved human hepatocytes can be used as an in vitro tool to study the induction of cytochrome P450 enzymes.**

Ans. **True.**

48. **Olanzapine is less likely to cause diabetes than conventional antipsychotics.**

Ans. **False.** More likely.

49. **More-hydrophilic β-adrenergic antagonists are more effective than the more-lipophilic ones for the treatment of akathisia.**

Ans. **False.** More-lipophilic ones are more effective.

50. **Atomoxetine should not be prescribed in combination with MAOIs.**

Ans. **True.**

Paper 13

		True	False
1.	Cigarette smoking induces hepatic CYP1A2.	☐	☐
2.	The risperidone molecule has a hydroxyl group for esterification making it not feasible for an oil-based delivery system.	☐	☐
3.	Dextroamphetamine has a higher incidence of cardiac side effects compared to methylphenidate.	☐	☐
4.	Prenatal exposure to tricyclic antidepressants has been associated with significant risk of congenital malformations.	☐	☐
5.	Phosphorylated proteins are known as third messengers.	☐	☐
6.	'Plasma membrane transporter' retransports the neurotransmitter into presynaptic nerve terminal.	☐	☐
7.	Rehospitalisation rates are lower with depot conventional antipsychotics than with their oral equivalents.	☐	☐
8.	Low-dose antipsychotic drugs have shown some efficacy in the treatment of cluster A personality disorders (DSM-1V).	☐	☐
9.	Alcohol inhibits the conversion of paracetamol to hepatotoxic derivatives.	☐	☐
10.	Monoamine oxidase inhibitors cause phenytoin toxicity by blocking phenytoin metabolism.	☐	☐
11.	Why a drug is ineffective when given orally but potent when given intravenously can be explained by the drug's first pass effects.	☐	☐
12.	Valproic acid inhibits the activities of both GABA ketoglutarate transaminase and succinic semialdehyde dehydrogenase (SSAD).	☐	☐
13.	Hyperventilation is more sensitive than lactate provocation in inducing panic attacks.	☐	☐
14.	Antagonism of tryptamine induced behavioural effects in rats was shown to be associated with binding affinity for the $5HT_2$ receptor.	☐	☐
15.	Aqueous-based injections are relatively less painful than oil-based injections.	☐	☐
16.	Captopril reduces the risk of bone marrow suppression when combined with clozapine.	☐	☐
17.	High-potency conventional antipsychotics have increased risk of teratogenicity.	☐	☐
18.	Two dosage forms of the same drug with an equal bioavailability are not necessarily bioequivalent.	☐	☐
19.	Sulpiride is not metabolized by the P450 enzymes.	☐	☐
20.	Whole body autoradiography is used in studying the distribution of the drug.	☐	☐
21.	Spontaneous remission is seen in approximately a quarter of patients with tardive dyskinesia.	☐	☐
22.	Benzodiazepines (BDZs) can be given safely along with acetazolamide in high altitudes.	☐	☐

	True	False

23. Monoamine neurotransmitters are transported from the cytoplasm into vesicles by vesicular monoamine transporter (VMAT). ☐ ☐

24. Reboxetine is a potent inhibitor of P450 enzymes. ☐ ☐

25. Carbamazepine blocks sodium channels in most brain regions. ☐ ☐

26. Loss of initial successful response to antidepressant treatment after several months of treatment is known as tachyphylaxis. ☐ ☐

27. Inhibition of amphetamine and cocaine induced agitation by a drug reflects central D_2 antagonism. ☐ ☐

28. Leptin induces insulin secretion. ☐ ☐

29. Neuroleptic malignant syndrome appears late in the course of neuroleptic treatment. ☐ ☐

30. Acetaldehyde is the first metabolite of alcohol. ☐ ☐

31. Tetrabenazine inhibits VMAT2 (vesicular monoamine transporter) activity. ☐ ☐

32. Lithium is contraindicated in liver disease. ☐ ☐

33. Length of treatment with drugs in social phobia should be at least 12 weeks. ☐ ☐

34. Weight gain is very rare with tranylcypromine. ☐ ☐

35. Caffeine can increase clozapine serum levels. ☐ ☐

36. Carbamazepine increases calcium influx into glial cells by its inhibitory effects on the peripheral benzodiazepine receptors. ☐ ☐

37. Temporary mild growth suppression is more likely with amphetamine treatment than with methylpheridate treatment for ADHD. ☐ ☐

38. Pimozide is contraindicated in patients with congenital long QT syndrome. ☐ ☐

39. Benzodiazepines have been reported to be effective in treating 'restless legs syndrome' that occurs during sleep. ☐ ☐

40. 'Median toxic dose' (TD50) of a drug is the dose at which 50% of patients have a therapeutic effect. ☐ ☐

41. Steady-state plasma concentrations of risperidone are reached after four long-acting injections. ☐ ☐

42. Amisulpiride is contraindicated in liver disease. ☐ ☐

43. Stimulants should be considered drugs of first choice in children with comorbid conduct and attention-deficit hyperactivity disorders with high aggression. ☐ ☐

44. Pre existing bundle-branch block increases the risk of experiencing cardiac side-effects induced by tricyclic antidepressants. ☐ ☐

45. Akathisia occurs in 10 to 20 percent of patients receiving metoclopramide. ☐ ☐

46. Benzodiazepines metabolized by glucuronide conjugation are not affected by cimetidine. ☐ ☐

47. Topiramate induced weight loss has been reported to be dose-related. ☐ ☐

	True	False
48. Tolerance to stimulants commonly develops in ADHD.	☐	☐
49. Desmopressin acetate (DDAVP) has been shown to be effective in the treatment of enuresis.	☐	☐
50. The distribution of a drug to the brain is determined by the blood-brain barrier but not by the brain's regional blood flow.	☐	☐

1. **Cigarette smoking induces hepatic CYP1A2.**

Ans. **True.**

2. **The risperidone molecule has a hydroxyl group for esterification making it not feasible for an oil-based delivery system.**

Ans. **False.** It does not have a hydroxyl group.

3. **Dextroamphetamine has a higher incidence of cardiac side effects compared to methylphenidate.**

Ans. **True.** For example tachycardia and hypertension.

4. **Prenatal exposure to tricyclic antidepressants has been associated with significant risk of congenital malformations.**

Ans. **False.**

5. **Phosphorylated proteins are known as third messengers.**

Ans. **True.**

6. **'Plasma membrane transporter' retransports the neurotransmitter into presynaptic nerve terminal.**

Ans. **True.**

7. **Rehospitalisation rates are lower with depot conventional antipsychotics than with their oral equivalents.**

Ans. **True.**

8. **Low-dose antipsychotic drugs have shown some efficacy in the treatment of cluster A personality disorders (DSM-1V).**

Ans. **True.**

9. **Alcohol inhibits the conversion of paracetamol to hepatotoxic derivatives.**

Ans. **False.** Alcohol stimulates the conversion.

10. **Monoamine oxidase inhibitors cause phenytoin toxicity by blocking phenytoin metabolism.**

Ans. **True.**

11. **Why a drug is ineffective when given orally but potent when given intravenously can be explained by the drug's first pass effects.**

Ans. **True.**

12. **Valproic acid inhibits the activities of both GABA ketoglutarate transaminase and succinic semialdehyde dehydrogenase (SSAD).**

Ans. **True.**

13. **Hyperventilation is more sensitive than lactate provocation in inducing panic attacks.**

Ans. **False.** It is less sensitive.

14. **Antagonism of tryptamine induced behavioural effects in rats was shown to be associated with binding affinity for the $5HT_2$ receptor.**

Ans. **True.**

15. **Aqueous-based injections are relatively less painful than oil-based injections.**

Ans. **True.**

16. **Captopril reduces the risk of bone marrow suppression when combined with clozapine.**

Ans. **False.** It increases the risk.

17. **High-potency conventional antipsychotics have increased risk of teratogenicity.**

Ans. **False.**

18. Two dosage forms of the same drug with an equal bioavailability are not necessarily bioequivalent.

Ans. True.

19. Sulpiride is not metabolized by the P450 enzymes.

Ans. True.

20. Whole body autoradiography is used in studying the distribution of the drug.

Ans. True.

21. Spontaneous remission is seen in approximately a quarter of patients with tardive dyskinesia.

Ans. True.

22. Benzodiazepines (BDZs) can be given safely along with acetazolamide in high altitudes.

Ans. False. BDZs antagonize the therapeutic effects of acetazolamide.

23. Monoamine neurotransmitters are transported from the cytoplasm into vesicles by vesicular monoamine transporter (VMAT).

Ans. True.

24. Reboxetine is a potent inhibitor of P450 enzymes.

Ans. False. It is devoid of any major inhibitory / inducing effects.

25. Carbamazepine blocks sodium channels in most brain regions.

Ans. True.

26. Loss of initial successful response to antidepressant treatment after several months of treatment is known as tachyphylaxis.

Ans. True.

27. Inhibition of amphetamine and cocaine induced agitation by a drug reflects central D_2 antagonism.

Ans. True.

28. Leptin induces insulin secretion.

Ans. False. Inhibits.

29. Neuroleptic malignant syndrome appears late in the course of neuroleptic treatment.

Ans. False.

30. Acetaldehyde is the first metabolite of alcohol.

Ans. True.

31. Tetrabenazine inhibits VMAT2 (vesicular monoamine transporter) activity.

Ans. True.

32. Lithium is contraindicated in liver disease.

Ans. False.

33. Length of treatment with drugs in social phobia should be at least 12 weeks.

Ans. True.

34. Weight gain is very rare with tranylcypromine.

Ans. True.

35. Caffeine can increase clozapine serum levels.

Ans. True. Caffeine is a substrate of the CYP1A2.

36. Carbamazepine increases calcium influx into glial cells by its inhibitory effects on the peripheral benzodiazepine receptors.

Ans. False. It reduces calcium influx.

37. **Temporary mild growth suppression is more likely with amphetamine treatment than with methylpheridate treatment for ADHD.**

Ans. **True.**

38. **Pimozide is contraindicated in patients with congenital long QT syndrome.**

Ans. **True.**

39. **Benzodiazepines have been reported to be effective in treating 'restless legs syndrome' that occurs during sleep.**

Ans. **True.**

40. **'Median toxic dose' (TD50) of a drug is the dose at which 50% of patients have a therapeutic effect.**

Ans. **False.** It is the does at which 50% experience a toxic effect.

41. **Steady-state plasma concentrations of risperidone are reached after four long-acting injections.**

Ans. **True.**

42. **Amisulpiride is contraindicated in liver disease.**

Ans. **False.**

43. **Stimulants should be considered drugs of first choice in children with comorbid conduct and attention-deficit hyperactivity disorders with high aggression.**

Ans. **True.**

44. **Pre existing bundle-branch block increases the risk of experiencing cardiac side-effects induced by tricyclic antidepressants.**

Ans. **True.**

45. **Akathisia occurs in 10 to 20 percent of patients receiving metoclopramide.**

Ans. **True.**

46. **Benzodiazepines metabolized by glucuronide conjugation are not affected by cimetidine.**

Ans. **True.**

47. **Topiramate induced weight loss has been reported to be dose-related.**

Ans. **True.**

48. **Tolerance to stimulants commonly develops in ADHD.**

Ans. **False.** This develops rarely.

49. **Desmopressin acetate (DDAVP) has been shown to be effective in the treatment of enuresis.**

Ans. **True.**

50. **The distribution of a drug to the brain is determined by the blood-brain barrier but not by the brain's regional blood flow.**

Ans. **False.** It is determined by both factors.

Paper 14

Questions

1. A drug which has a therapeutic window shows a curvilinear dose-response curve.

2. Elevated white blood cell count is seen in neuroleptic malignant syndrome but not in lethal catatonia.

3. Flumazenil (benzodiazepine antagonist) can, very rarely, cause convulsions.

4. CYP1A2-inducing capacity of cigarette smoking is weaker than its CYP3A4-inducing capacity.

5. Carbamazepine has suppressing effects on limbic kindling.

6. More than 50% of patients with Tourette's disorder respond favourably to either haloperidol or pimozide.

7. 'Periodic limb movement disorder' that occurs during sleep can be treated by benzodiazepines.

8. A drug's toxicity or safety is determined by its ratio of the median toxic dose (TD50) to the median effective dose (ED50).

9. Non-depolazing muscle relaxants have a faster onset of action than suxamethonium.

10. Methylpheridate can cause a transient rise in intraocular pressure which is not associated with closure of the angle.

11. 'Median effective dose' (ED50) of a drug is the dose at which 50% of patients have a therapeutic effect.

12. 'Idiosyncratic reaction' to a drug can be defined as a genetically determined abnormal reactivity.

13. Methadone has longer half-life than L-α-acetylmethadol hydrochloride (LAAM).

14. Side-effects of clonidine include Raynaud's phenomenon.

15. Buprenorphine is a partial μ-opioid agonist.

16. Selegiline is a selective MAO-B inhibitor at high doses.

17. In men, the symptoms of hyperprolactinaemia include impotence.

18. A 'synergistic effect' describes the combined effect of two drugs that is equal to the sum of the effect of each agent given alone.

19. Activated charcoal interrupts the enterohepatic circulation of tricyclic antidepressants.

20. Valproate can rarely cause acute haemorrhagic pancreatitis.

21. M-chlorophenylpiperazine is an active metabolite of trazodone.

22. Opiate antagonists are useful in diagnosing physical dependence on opioid drugs.

23. 6-β-naltrexol is an inactive metabolite of naltrexone.

24. The dissociation between inhibition of amphetamine-induced behaviour and induction of catalepsy is narrower with risperidone than with haloperidol.

25. Mirtazapine acts by antagonising α2-adrenergic auto-and heteroceptors and 5HT$_2$ and 5HT$_3$ receptors. ☐ ☐

26. LAAM (L-α-Acetylmethadol) has two major active metabolites nor-LAAM and dinor-LAAM. ☐ ☐

27. Carbamazepine increases the anticoagulant effect of warfarin. ☐ ☐

28. Absorption of drugs is severely affected in the elderly. ☐ ☐

29. Isocarboxazid is safer to use in moderate liver disease. ☐ ☐

30. The most common side-effect of clonidine is sedation. ☐ ☐

31. Hallucinations occur with parenteral doses of pentazocine above 60 mg. ☐ ☐

32. Clomethiazole is an antagonist at GABA-A receptor. ☐ ☐

33. If hepatic transaminase levels increase to more than three times normal, valproate should be discontinued. ☐ ☐

34. Bupropion has no effect on 5-HT uptake. ☐ ☐

35. Tolerance develops to the antagonism of opioid effects after 6 weeks of naltrexone treatment. ☐ ☐

36. Prolactin is encoded by a single gene in chromosome 6. ☐ ☐

37. Co-administration of valproate with aspirin reduces the free fraction of valproate. ☐ ☐

38. Naloxone is an intravenous analogue of naltrexone and a non-selective opioid antagonist. ☐ ☐

39. Glucuronide conjugation and hepatic oxidative metabolism of drugs are deficient in neonates. ☐ ☐

40. Aspirin improves cognitive function in vascular dementia. ☐ ☐

41. Phenytoin reduces quetiapine clearance. ☐ ☐

42. An 'additive effect' is one in which the combined effect of two drugs is equal to the sum of the effect of each agent given alone. ☐ ☐

43. Hydroxybupropion is an inactive metabolite of bupropion. ☐ ☐

44. Protein binding is reduced in elderly people. ☐ ☐

45. Drugs which are more water-soluble are poorly dialysed. ☐ ☐

46. The hydroxylation of diazepam is reduced in the newborn. ☐ ☐

47. The placental transfer of drugs is related to their lipophilicity and low molecular weight. ☐ ☐

48. 'Sternbach diagnostic criteria' are used to classify the 'neuroleptic malignant syndrome'. ☐ ☐

49. Naltrexone blocks endogenous opioid peptides in addition to injected opioid drugs. ☐ ☐

50. Fluvoxamine increases the anticoagulant effect of warfarin. ☐ ☐

Paper 14

1. A drug which has a therapeutic window shows a curvilinear dose-response curve.
Ans. True.

2. Elevated white blood cell count is seen in neuroleptic malignant syndrome but not in lethal catatonia.
Ans. True.

3. Flumazenil (benzodiazepine antagonist) can, very rarely, cause convulsions.
Ans. True.

4. CYP1A2-inducing capacity of cigarette smoking is weaker than its CYP3A4 -inducing capacity.
Ans. False. It is stronger.

5. Carbamazepine has suppressing effects on limbic kindling.
Ans. True.

6. More than 50% of patients with Tourette's disorder respond favourably to either haloperidol or pimozide.
Ans. True.

7. 'Periodic limb movement disorder' that occurs during sleep can be treated by benzodiazepines.
Ans. True.

8. A drug's toxicity or safety is determined by its ratio of the median toxic dose (TD50) to the median effective dose (ED50).
Ans. True.

9. Non-depolazing muscle relaxants have a faster onset of action than suxamethonium.
Ans. False. They have a slower onset of action.

10. Methylpheridate can cause a transient rise in intraocular pressure which is not associated with closure of the angle.
Ans. True.

11. 'Median effective dose' (ED50) of a drug is the dose at which 50% of patients have a therapeutic effect.
Ans. True.

12. 'Idiosyncratic reaction' to a drug can be defined as a genetically determined abnormal reactivity.
Ans. True.

13. Methadone has longer half-life than L-α-acetylmethadol hydrochloride (LAAM).
Ans. False. It has a shorter half-life (methadone = 25 hr, LAAM = 2-4 days).

14. Side-effects of clonidine include Raynaud's phenomenon.
Ans. True.

15. Buprenorphine is a partial μ-opioid agonist.
Ans. True.

16. Selegiline is a selective MAO-B inhibitor at high doses.
Ans. False. At lower doses.

17. In men, the symptoms of hyperprolactinaemia include impotence.
Ans. True.

18. A 'synergistic effect' describes the combined effect of two drugs that is equal to the sum of the effect of each agent given alone.
Ans. False. It is where the combined effect is greater than the sum of the effects.

19. Activated charcoal interrupts the enterohepatic circulation of tricyclic antidepressants.

Ans. True.

20. Valproate can rarely cause acute haemorrhagic pancreatitis.

Ans. True.

21. M-chlorophenylpiperazine is an active metabolite of trazodone.

Ans. True.

22. Opiate antagonists are useful in diagnosing physical dependence on opioid drugs.

Ans. True.

23. 6-β-naltrexol is an inactive metabolite of naltrexone.

Ans. False. It is active.

24. The dissociation between inhibition of amphetamine-induced behaviour and induction of catalepsy is narrower with risperidone than with haloperidol.

Ans. False. It is wider.

25. Mirtazapine acts by antagonising α2-adrenergic auto-and heteroceptors and $5HT_2$ and $5HT_3$ receptors.

Ans. True.

26. LAAM (L-α-Acetylmethadol) has two major active metabolites nor-LAAM and dinor-LAAM.

Ans. True.

27. Carbamazepine increases the anticoagulant effect of warfarin.

Ans. False. Reduces the effect by increasing the metabolism of warfarin.

28. Absorption of drugs is severely affected in the elderly.

Ans. False.

29. Isocarboxazid is safer to use in moderate liver disease.

Ans. False. It is contraindicated.

30. The most common side-effect of clonidine is sedation.

Ans. True.

31. Hallucinations occur with parenteral doses of pentazocine above 60 mg.

Ans. True.

32. Clomethiazole is an antagonist at GABA-A receptor.

Ans. False. It is an agonist.

33. If hepatic transaminase levels increase to more than three times normal, valproate should be discontinued.

Ans. True.

34. Bupropion has no effect on 5-HT uptake.

Ans. True.

35. Tolerance develops to the antagonism of opioid effects after 6 weeks of naltrexone treatment.

Ans. False.

36. Prolactin is encoded by a single gene in chromosome 6.

Ans. True.

37. Co-administration of valproate with aspirin reduces the free fraction of valproate.

Ans. False. Increases.

38. Naloxone is an intravenous analogue of naltrexone and a non-selective opioid antagonist.

Ans. True.

39. **Glucuronide conjugation and hepatic oxidative metabolism of drugs are deficient in neonates.**
Ans. **True.**

40. **Aspirin improves cognitive function in vascular dementia.**
Ans. **True.**

41. **Phenytoin reduces quetiapine clearance.**
Ans. **False.** Increases.

42. **An 'additive effect' is one in which the combined effect of two drugs is equal to the sum of the effect of each agent given alone.**
Ans. **True.**

43. **Hydroxybupropion is an inactive metabolite of bupropion.**
Ans. **False.** It is an active metabolite.

44. **Protein binding is reduced in elderly people.**
Ans. **True.**

45. **Drugs which are more water-soluble are poorly dialysed.**
Ans. **False.** More water soluble drugs are better dialysed.

46. **The hydroxylation of diazepam is reduced in the newborn.**
Ans. **True.**

47. **The placental transfer of drugs is related to their lipophilicity and low molecular weight.**
Ans. **True.**

48. **'Sternbach diagnostic criteria' are used to classify the 'neuroleptic malignant syndrome'.**
Ans. **False.** It us used in serotonin syndrome.

49. **Naltrexone blocks endogenous opioid peptides in addition to injected opioid drugs.**
Ans. **True.**

50. **Fluvoxamine increases the anticoagulant effect of warfarin.**
Ans. **True.** By inhibiting the hepatic metabolism of warfarin.

Paper 15

		True	False
1.	Following birth, both glomerular filtration rate and tubular function take about 6 weeks to reach adult levels.	☐	☐
2.	Coadministration of phenytoin and rifampicin reduces the phenytoin effects.	☐	☐
3.	The tricyclic antidepressants prevent the reuptake of noradrenaline into peripheral adrenergic neurones.	☐	☐
4.	Dietary salt-restriction leads to reduced serum lithium levels.	☐	☐
5.	Excessive coffee-intake causes a reduction in serum lithium levels.	☐	☐
6.	Coadministration of lamotrigine with valproate significantly increases the half-life of lamotrigine.	☐	☐
7.	Protein binding is increased in neonates.	☐	☐
8.	Inter-individual variation in drugs metabolism is more in younger than in elderly patients.	☐	☐
9.	Concurrent use of lithium carbonate and potassium iodide may increase the risk of hypothyroidism.	☐	☐
10.	The larger the drug molecule, the lower the rate of clearance by dialysis.	☐	☐
11.	Acamprosate does not interact with alcohol or disulfiram.	☐	☐
12.	Lithium induced neutrophil leucocytosis is irreversible.	☐	☐
13.	People with first-episode schizophrenia show a greater response to neuroleptic treatment than chronic subjects.	☐	☐
14.	Flupenthixol and fluphenazine depot antipsychotic injections are associated with weight gain.	☐	☐
15.	Caffeine can prolong ECT-induced seizures.	☐	☐
16.	5-HT depletion exacerbates symptoms in people with untreated OCD.	☐	☐
17.	Lithium carbonate has known efficacy in the treatment of cluster headaches.	☐	☐
18.	Mortality due to neuroleptic malignant syndrome is 20%.	☐	☐
19.	The purpose of continuation treatment with antidepressant drugs is the prevention of relapse.	☐	☐
20.	The purpose of maintenance treatment with antidepressant drugs is the prevention of recurrence of a new episode after full recovery.	☐	☐
21.	D2 receptor occupancy of antipsychotic drugs can be estimated by using positron emission tomography with (^{11}C) N-methylspiperone.	☐	☐
22.	Individuals with first-episode schizophrenia are less sensitive to extrapyramidal symptoms.	☐	☐
23.	The dextrorotatory isomer of fenfluramine can be used as an adjunct to dietary restriction in the treatment of drug-induced obesity.	☐	☐
24.	Periodic limb movement disorder can be worsened by MAOI antidepressants.	☐	☐

25. Dialysis is of no use in treatment of tricyclic antidepressant poisoning as the drugs are highly protein bound. ☐ ☐

26. Diazepam has less anticonvulsant properties than chlordiazepoxide. ☐ ☐

27. Drugs which are more protein bound are poorly cleared by dialysis. ☐ ☐

28. Antiparkinsonian drugs alter the absorption of antipsychotic drugs. ☐ ☐

29. Antidepressant drug treatment, at an effective dose, should be maintained for a period of 4-6 months following acute symptoms resolution. ☐ ☐

30. Volume of distribution for lithium decreases in older patients. ☐ ☐

31. Anti-inflammatory drugs can be used to treat Alzheimer's disease. ☐ ☐

32. Phenelzine is effective in treatment of patients with social phobia. ☐ ☐

33. Dantrolene reduces muscle rigidity in the treatment of neuroleptic malignant syndrome. ☐ ☐

34. Single-dose kinetic studies for high-clearance drugs are adequate to exclude the possibility of altered pharmacokinetics in elderly. ☐ ☐

35. Clozapine often results in continuous weight gain. ☐ ☐

36. Benzodiazepine inverse agonists have anxiogenic activity. ☐ ☐

37. Antipsychotic drugs decrease neurotensin (a tridecapeptide) concentrations in the nucleus accumbens. ☐ ☐

38. Buccofacial dyskinesia is a rare side-effect of modafinil. ☐ ☐

39. Diazepam can cause paradoxical increase in aggression. ☐ ☐

40. Naturalistic studies have shown that tricyclic antidepressants are often prescribed at higher doses. ☐ ☐

41. Radiolabelled carfentanil is used as a ligand to study central benzodiazepine receptors. ☐ ☐

42. Loss of weight is a recognised symptom of benzodiazepine withdrawal syndrome. ☐ ☐

43. Adipsic hypernatremia can be caused by severe depression. ☐ ☐

44. Lithium may be associated with prolonged muscle paralysis during ECT. ☐ ☐

45. Coadministration of neuroleptic and tricyclic antidepressant is likely to prolong the activity of both drugs. ☐ ☐

46. Flumazenil blocks the effects of benzodiazepine agonists but not inverse agonists. ☐ ☐

47. Hyperprolactinemia is associated with increased risk for bone loss. ☐ ☐

48. Volume of distribution (Vd) increases for lipid-soluble drugs and decreases for water-soluble drugs in elderly people. ☐ ☐

49. Overdose of bromocriptine can present with severe hypertension and psychosis. ☐ ☐

50. Carbamazepine and valproate can be used by women who are breastfeeding. ☐ ☐

Paper 15

1. Following birth, both glomerular filtration rate and tubular function take about 6 weeks to reach adult levels.

Ans. **False.** It takes 6 months.

2. Coadministration of phenytoin and rifampicin reduces the phenytoin effects.

Ans. **True.** Rifampicin is an enzyme inducing drug.

3. The tricyclic antidepressants prevent the reuptake of noradrenaline into peripheral adrenergic neurones.

Ans. **True.**

4. Dietary salt-restriction leads to reduced serum lithium levels.

Ans. **False.** It leads to increased serum lithium levels.

5. Excessive coffee-intake causes a reduction in serum lithium levels.

Ans. **True.**

6. Coadministration of lamotrigine with valproate significantly increases the half-life of lamotrigine.

Ans. **True.**

7. Protein binding is increased in neonates.

Ans. **False.** It is reduced.

8. Inter-individual variation in drugs metabolism is more in younger than in elderly patients.

Ans. **False.** There is greater variation in the elderly.

9. Concurrent use of lithium carbonate and potassium iodide may increase the risk of hypothyroidism.

Ans. **True.**

10. The larger the drug molecule, the lower the rate of clearance by dialysis.

Ans. **True.**

11. Acamprosate does not interact with alcohol or disulfiram.

Ans. **True.**

12. Lithium induced neutrophil leucocytosis is irreversible.

Ans. **False.**

13. People with first-episode schizophrenia show a greater response to neuroleptic treatment than chronic subjects.

Ans. **True.**

14. Flupenthixol and fluphenazine depot antipsychotic injections are associated with weight gain.

Ans. **True.**

15. Caffeine can prolong ECT-induced seizures.

Ans. **True.**

16. 5-HT depletion exacerbates symptoms in people with untreated OCD.

Ans. **False.**

17. Lithium carbonate has known efficacy in the treatment of cluster headaches.

Ans. **True.**

18. Mortality due to neuroleptic malignant syndrome is 20%.

Ans. **True.**

19. The purpose of continuation treatment with antidepressant drugs is the prevention of relapse.
Ans. True.

20. The purpose of maintenance treatment with antidepressant drugs is the prevention of recurrence of a new episode after full recovery.
Ans. True.

21. D2 receptor occupancy of antipsychotic drugs can be estimated by using positron emission tomography with (^{11}C) N-methylspiperone.
Ans. False. (^{11}C) raclopride is used.

22. Individuals with first-episode schizophrenia are less sensitive to extrapyramidal symptoms.
Ans. False. They are more sensitive.

23. The dextrorotatory isomer of fenfluramine can be used as an adjunct to dietary restriction in the treatment of drug-induced obesity.
Ans. True.

24. Periodic limb movement disorder can be worsened by MAOI antidepressants.
Ans. True.

25. Dialysis is of no use in treatment of tricyclic antidepressant poisoning as the drugs are highly protein bound.
Ans. True.

26. Diazepam has less anticonvulsant properties than chlordiazepoxide.
Ans. False. It has more.

27. Drugs which are more protein bound are poorly cleared by dialysis.
Ans. True.

28. Antiparkinsonian drugs alter the absorption of antipsychotic drugs.
Ans. True. By changing gut motility.

29. Antidepressant drug treatment, at an effective dose, should be maintained for a period of 4 – 6 months following acute symptoms resolution.
Ans. True.

30. Volume of distribution for lithium decreases in older patients.
Ans. True.

31. Anti-inflammatory drugs can be used to treat Alzheimer's disease.
Ans. False.

32. Phenelzine is effective in treatment of patients with social phobia.
Ans. True.

33. Dantrolene reduces muscle rigidity in the treatment of neuroleptic malignant syndrome.
Ans. True.

34. Single-dose kinetic studies for high-clearance drugs are adequate to exclude the possibility of altered pharmacokinetics in elderly.
Ans. False. Multiple-dose kinetic studies are essential.

35. Clozapine often results in continuous weight gain.
Ans. True.

36. Benzodiazepine inverse agonists have anxiogenic activity.
Ans. True.

37. Antipsychotic drugs decrease neurotensin (a tridecapeptide) concentrations in the nucleus accumbens.
Ans. True.

38. **Buccofacial dyskinesia is a rare side-effect of modafinil.**

Ans. True.

39. **Diazepam can cause paradoxical increase in aggression.**

Ans. True.

40. **Naturalistic studies have shown that tricyclic antidepressants are often prescribed at higher doses.**

Ans. False.

41. **Radiolabelled carfentanil is used as a ligand to study central benzodiazepine receptors.**

Ans. False. To study opiate receptors.

42. **Loss of weight is a recognised symptom of benzodiazepine withdrawal syndrome.**

Ans. True.

43. **Adipsic hypernatremia can be caused by severe depression.**

Ans. True.

44. **Lithium may be associated with prolonged muscle paralysis during ECT.**

Ans. True. It interferes with pseudocholinesterase.

45. **Coadministration of neuroleptic and tricyclic antidepressant is likely to prolong the activity of both drugs.**

Ans. True.

46. **Flumazenil blocks the effects of benzodiazepine agonists but not inverse agonists.**

Ans. False. It blocks both.

47. **Hyperprolactinemia is associated with increased risk for bone loss.**

Ans. True.

48. **Volume of distribution (Vd) increases for lipid-soluble drugs and decreases for water-soluble drugs in elderly people.**

Ans. True.

49. **Overdose of bromocriptine can present with severe hypertension and psychosis.**

Ans. False. It causes severe hypotension and psychosis.

50. **Carbamazepine and valproate can be used by women who are breastfeeding.**

Ans. True.

Paper 16

		True	False
1.	Tardive dyskinesia is not painful.	☐	☐
2.	Maintenance therapy with lithium for bipolar disorder patients significantly reduces suicide risk.	☐	☐
3.	Onset of tardive dyskinesia in older patients is high but not rapid.	☐	☐
4.	Benzodiazepine receptors BZ_2 are mainly found in hippocampus and neocortex.	☐	☐
5.	A lower ratio of mg of drug to kg of body weight should be used in children.	☐	☐
6.	Overdose of bupropion can cause hallucinations and seizures.	☐	☐
7.	Fluoxetine may cause weight loss during the initial phase of the treatment.	☐	☐
8.	Half-life of a drug is inversely proportional to its volume of distribution.	☐	☐
9.	Elevated plasma non-esterified fatty acids (NEFA) are associated with insulin resistance caused by some antipsychotic drugs.	☐	☐
10.	Loss of sensitivity to a drug represents a rightward shift of the dose-effect curve.	☐	☐
11.	Benzodiazepines have been reported to diminish the effectiveness of unilateral ECT.	☐	☐
12.	Discontinuation of antipsychotic drugs can cause cholinergic rebound.	☐	☐
13.	Propofol is a short acting drug used for induction and maintenance of anaesthesia for ECT.	☐	☐
14.	Therapeutic action of neuroleptic drugs may be increased by concurrent use of antiparkinsonian drugs.	☐	☐
15.	Non-MAOI and non-tricyclic antidepressants are relatively safe in overdose.	☐	☐
16.	Cytochrome P450 isoenzyme CYP 3A4 activity is greater in younger women than in men and postmenopausal women.	☐	☐
17.	Long term administration of antipsychotic drugs leads to 'depolarization block' of dopamine cells.	☐	☐
18.	The free or unbound percentage of albumin-bound drugs decreases with age.	☐	☐
19.	'Nootropics' are cyclic analogues of GABA and structurally related to piracetam.	☐	☐
20.	Lithium may increase parathyroid hormone levels.	☐	☐
21.	Fenfluramine has been associated with valvular heart disease.	☐	☐
22.	Coadministration of an SSRI and a tricyclic antidepressant reduces the levels of tricyclic antidepressant.	☐	☐
23.	L-tryptophan should not be given with an SSRI.	☐	☐
24.	SSRIs cause more impairment than TCAs on critical flicker fusion test.	☐	☐
25.	The syndrome of inappropriate antidiuretic hormone secretion (SIADH) has been associated with treatment with fluoxetine in older patients.	☐	☐

26. Sibutramine is a β-phenylethylamine that inhibits the reuptake of serotonin and norepinephrine and is used for the treatment of obesity. ☐ ☐

27. Tricyclic antidepressant-induced ECG changes include a decrease in T wave amplitude. ☐ ☐

28. Therapeutic index in relation to acute extrapyramidal side-effects is wider with haloperidol than with olanzapine. ☐ ☐

29. 5HT2a antagonists have shown anti-akathisia properties in some patients. ☐ ☐

30. QTc is a rate-corrected interval, which is adjusted to take account of changes in the heart rate. ☐ ☐

31. Cholecystokinin receptor 'CCK-B' antagonists demonstrate anxiolytic properties. ☐ ☐

32. Venlafaxine in higher doses is associated with hypotension. ☐ ☐

33. Cardiovascular side-effects of tricyclic antidepressants are dose related. ☐ ☐

34. Tetrabenazine blocks the action of reserpine. ☐ ☐

35. EC_{50} means the concentration of a drug evoking a half maximal response. ☐ ☐

36. Adherence to antipsychotic drugs is better if the 'subjective' response to the medication is slow. ☐ ☐

37. Iron-deficiency anaemia may cause akathisia that is identical in phenomenology to neuroleptic-induced akathisia. ☐ ☐

38. NICE guidance on atypical antipsychotics states that atypical and typical antipsychotics should not be prescribed together except during changeover of medication. ☐ ☐

39. The specific location of COMT gene is on the long arm of chromosome 22 at 22q11.21. ☐ ☐

40. Treatment with clozapine is associated with increased risk of dyslipidemia. ☐ ☐

41. Lamotrigine does not induce mania in patients with bipolar disorder. ☐ ☐

42. Drugs that inhibit CYP1A2 can precipitate caffeine toxicity. ☐ ☐

43. Toxicity from highly protein bound drugs is less common in patients with hepatic impairment. ☐ ☐

44. Acid urine decreases ionization of basic drugs. ☐ ☐

45. Plasma levels of an antipsychotic drug released from regular depot injection rise over several treatment cycles after initiation, without increasing the given dose. ☐ ☐

46. Zuclopenthixol acetate should not be given as intramuscular injection to neuroleptic naïve patients. ☐ ☐

47. Chlorpromazine is less associated with diabetes than haloperidol. ☐ ☐

48. Clozapine does not cause galactorrhea. ☐ ☐

49. Benzodiazepine withdrawal syndrome may worsen with buspirone. ☐ ☐

50. Neurotensin is colocalized with dopamine in the mesolimbic dopamine pathway. ☐ ☐

1. Tardive dyskinesia is not painful.
Ans. True.

2. Maintenance therapy with lithium for bipolar disorder patients significantly reduces suicide risk.
Ans. True.

3. Onset of tardive dyskinesia in older patients is high but not rapid.
Ans. False. Rapid and high incidence.

4. Benzodiazepine receptors BZ_2 are mainly found in hippocampus and neocortex.
Ans. True.

5. A lower ratio of mg of drug to kg of body weight should be used in children.
Ans. False. A higher ratio should be used.

6. Overdose of bupropion can cause hallucinations and seizures.
Ans. True.

7. Fluoxetine may cause weight loss during the initial phase of the treatment.
Ans. True.

8. Half-life of a drug is inversely proportional to its volume of distribution.
Ans. False. They are directly proportional.

9. Elevated plasma non-esterified fatty acids (NEFA) are associated with insulin resistance caused by some antipsychotic drugs.
Ans. True.

10. Loss of sensitivity to a drug represents a rightward shift of the dose-effect curve.
Ans. True.

11. Benzodiazepines have been reported to diminish the effectiveness of unilateral ECT.
Ans. True.

12. Discontinuation of antipsychotic drugs can cause cholinergic rebound.
Ans. True.

13. Propofol is a short acting drug used for induction and maintenance of anaesthesia for ECT.
Ans. True.

14. Therapeutic action of neuroleptic drugs may be increased by concurrent use of antiparkinsonian drugs.
Ans. False. This reduces the effect.

15. Non-MAOI and non-tricyclic antidepressants are relatively safe in overdose.
Ans. True.

16. Cytochrome P450 isoenzyme CYP 3A4 activity is greater in younger women than in men and postmenopausal women.
Ans. True.

17. Long term administration of antipsychotic drugs leads to 'depolarization block' of dopamine cells.
Ans. True.

18. The free or unbound percentage of albumin-bound drugs decreases with age.
Ans. False. It increases.

19. 'Nootropics' are cyclic analogues of GABA and structurally related to piracetam.

Ans. **True.** They may also improve memory and learning.

20. Lithium may increase parathyroid hormone levels.

Ans. **True.**

21. Fenfluramine has been associated with valvular heart disease.

Ans. **True.**

22. Coadministration of an SSRI and a tricyclic antidepressant reduces the levels of tricyclic antidepressant.

Ans. **False.** It increases them.

23. L-tryptophan should not be given with an SSRI.

Ans. **True.**

24. SSRIs cause more impairment than TCAs on critical flicker fusion test.

Ans. **False.**

25. The syndrome of inappropriate antidiuretic hormone secretion (SIADH) has been associated with treatment with fluoxetine in older patients.

Ans. **True.**

26. Sibutramine is a β-phenylethylamine that inhibits the reuptake of serotonin and norepinephrine and is used for the treatment of obesity.

Ans. **True.**

27. Tricyclic antidepressant-induced ECG changes include a decrease in T wave amplitude.

Ans. **True.** They also include increased PR, QRS and QT intervals.

28. Therapeutic index in relation to acute extrapyramidal side-effects is wider with haloperidol than with olanzapine.

Ans. **False.** Haloperidol has a narrower index.

29. 5HT2a antagonists have shown anti-akathisia properties in some patients.

Ans. **True.** For example, mianserin, ritanserin and cyproheptadine.

30. QTc is a rate-corrected interval, which is adjusted to take account of changes in the heart rate.

Ans. **True.**

31. Cholecystokinin receptor 'CCK-B' antagonists demonstrate anxiolytic properties.

Ans. **True.**

32. Venlafaxine in higher doses is associated with hypotension.

Ans. **False.** It is associated with elevated blood pressure.

33. Cardiovascular side-effects of tricyclic antidepressants are dose related.

Ans. **True.**

34. Tetrabenazine blocks the action of reserpine.

Ans. **True.**

35. EC_{50} means the concentration of a drug evoking a half maximal response.

Ans. **True.**

36. Adherence to antipsychotic drugs is better if the 'subjective' response to the medication is slow.

Ans. **False.** Adherence is better if the response is rapid.

37. Iron-deficiency anaemia may cause akathisia that is identical in phenomenology to neuroleptic-induced akathisia.

Ans. **True.**

38. **NICE guidance on atypical antipsychotics states that atypical and typical antipsychotics should not be prescribed together except during changeover of medication.**
Ans. **True.**

39. **The specific location of COMT gene is on the long arm of chromosome 22 at 22q11.21.**
Ans. **True.**

40. **Treatment with clozapine is associated with increased risk of dyslipidemia.**
Ans. **True.**

41. **Lamotrigine does not induce mania in patients with bipolar disorder.**
Ans. **True.**

42. **Drugs that inhibit CYP1A2 can precipitate caffeine toxicity.**
Ans. **True.**

43. **Toxicity from highly protein bound drugs is less common in patients with hepatic impairment.**
Ans. **False.** It is more common in such patients.

44. **Acid urine decreases ionization of basic drugs.**
Ans. **False.** It increases this.

45. **Plasma levels of an antipsychotic drug released from regular depot injection rise over several treatment cycles after initiation, without increasing the given dose.**
Ans. **True.**

46. **Zuclopenthixol acetate should not be given as intramuscular injection to neuroleptic naïve patients.**
Ans. **True.**

47. **Chlorpromazine is less associated with diabetes than haloperidol.**
Ans. **False.** It is more associated with diabetes.

48. **Clozapine does not cause galactorrhea.**
Ans. **True.**

49. **Benzodiazepine withdrawal syndrome may worsen with buspirone.**
Ans. **False.**

50. **Neurotensin is colocalized with dopamine in the mesolimbic dopamine pathway.**
Ans. **True.**

Paper 17

	True	False
1. Biotransformation of a drug results in conversion of the drug into less polar molecules.	☐	☐
2. Benzodiazepines have been associated with an increased risk of road traffic accidents.	☐	☐
3. Clozapine is associated with hyperosmolar coma.	☐	☐
4. Risk factors for developing neuroleptic-induced parkinsonism include previous history of neuroleptic-induced parkinsonism.	☐	☐
5. Modafinil is indicated for the treatment of excessive daytime sleepiness associated with narcolepsy and contra-indicated in obstructive sleep apnoea.	☐	☐
6. Procyclidine is indicated for the treatment and symptomatic relief of all forms of Parkinson's disease.	☐	☐
7. Alkaline urine facilitates the excretion of acid drugs.	☐	☐
8. Plasma levels of a drug take less time to reach steady state levels in patients with hepatic impairment.	☐	☐
9. Impaired glucose tolerance in the absence of diabetes increases the risk of cardiovascular morbidity.	☐	☐
10. Structurally nonspecific drugs do not display stereoselectivity.	☐	☐
11. L-arginine is converted into nitric oxide and L-citruline by the enzyme nitric oxide hydroxylase.	☐	☐
12. Both demethylated and didemethylated metabolites of escitalopram are active.	☐	☐
13. Medication-induced movement disorders should be coded on Axis I DSM-IV.	☐	☐
14. Benzodiazepine receptor binding can be inhibited by large doses of caffeine.	☐	☐
15. Amisulpride has been associated with ketoacidosis.	☐	☐
16. Naloxone antagonism of diamorphine at opioid receptors is an example of 'competitive antagonism'.	☐	☐
17. Clozapine should not be used with propylthiouracil.	☐	☐
18. Parkinsonian tremors are finer and faster than non-parkinsonian tremors.	☐	☐
19. Risperidone does not affect the pharmacokinetic parameters of lithium.	☐	☐
20. Bromocriptine increases the plasma levels of growth hormone.	☐	☐
21. Coadministration of lithium and metronidazole increases risk of lithium toxicity.	☐	☐
22. Sodium valproate inhibits metabolism of phenytoin, carbamazepine and ethosuximide.	☐	☐
23. Pharmacokinetic interactions alter the plasma concentrations of the interacting drugs.	☐	☐
24. Treatment with olanzapine is associated with increased risk of dyslipidemia.	☐	☐

	True	False

25. Coadministration of omeprazole and escitalopram can result in reduced plasma concentrations of escitalopram. ☐ ☐

26. Neuroleptic-induced acute akathisia typically occurs within 4 weeks of initiating or increasing the dose of a neuroleptic medication. ☐ ☐

27. Propranolol increases plasma concentration of chlorpromazine. ☐ ☐

28. Sulpiride has a low affinity for dopamine receptors in the tubero infundibular tract. ☐ ☐

29. Antiphospholipid antibodies are associated with phenothiazines (e.g. chlorpromazine) in some patients. ☐ ☐

30. In functional antagonism two different agonists evoke opposing responses from a single biological system by activating different receptors. ☐ ☐

31. Bioavailability of mirtazapine is decreased by more than 50% when coadministered with cimetidine. ☐ ☐

32. Tissue tolerance to a drug is different from its metabolic tolerance. ☐ ☐

33. Up to two-thirds of depressed patients have a blunted thyrotropin (TSH) response to thyrotropin-releasing hormone (TRH). ☐ ☐

34. M-chlorophenylpiperazine is an inactive metabolite of trazodone. ☐ ☐

35. Tamoxifen (an oestrogen receptor antagonist used for the treatment of breast cancer) can induce depression. ☐ ☐

36. Lithium-induced fine postural tremor has a frequency between 8 and 12 cycles per second. ☐ ☐

37. Gabapentin does not have either active or inactive metabolites. ☐ ☐

38. The second-generation H_1 antagonist astemizole can cause prolongation of the QTc interval, resulting in polymorphic ventricular tachycardia (torsades de pointes). ☐ ☐

39. Low serum protein can result in greater sensitivity to conventional doses of lithium. ☐ ☐

40. Neuroleptic-induced parkinsonian tremor is a coarse, rhythmic, resting tremor with a frequency between 3 and 6 cycles per second. ☐ ☐

41. Benzodiazepine antagonists have no intrinsic activity themselves. ☐ ☐

42. Lamotrigine does not affect the metabolism of other drugs. ☐ ☐

43. Decreased prolactin levels may be seen following cocaine withdrawal. ☐ ☐

44. Clozapine can decrease platelet count. ☐ ☐

45. Severe agitation can cause myoglobunuria secondary to muscle breakdown. ☐ ☐

46. Risk of cardiac side effects due to tricyclic antidepressants is low when they are coadminstered with Type I antiarrhythmic drugs. ☐ ☐

47. Neuroleptic-induced acute dystonia occurs most commonly in young males. ☐ ☐

48. The demethyl metabolite of mirtazapine is pharmacologically inactive. ☐ ☐

	True	False
49. Inverse benzodiazepine agonists decrease the chloride channel openings and produce anxiety and convulsions.	☐	☐
50. Increased levels of serum salicylate can cause organic hallucinosis.	☐	☐

1. Biotransformation of a drug results in conversion of the drug into less polar molecules.
Ans. **False.** More polar molecules.

2. Benzodiazepines have been associated with an increased risk of road traffic accidents.
Ans. **True.**

3. Clozapine is associated with hyperosmolar coma.
Ans. **True.**

4. Risk factors for developing neuroleptic-induced parkinsonism include previous history of neuroleptic-induced parkinsonism.
Ans. **True.**

5. Modafinil is indicated for the treatment of excessive daytime sleepiness associated with narcolepsy and contra-indicated in obstructive sleep apnoea.
Ans. **False.** It is indicated in both.

6. Procyclidine is indicated for the treatment and symptomatic relief of all forms of Parkinson's disease.
Ans. **True.**

7. Alkaline urine facilitates the excretion of acid drugs.
Ans. **True.**

8. Plasma levels of a drug take less time to reach steady state levels in patients with hepatic impairment.
Ans. **False.** It takes longer in such patients.

9. Impaired glucose tolerance in the absence of diabetes increases the risk of cardiovascular morbidity.
Ans. **True.**

10. Structurally nonspecific drugs do not display stereoselectivity.
Ans. **True.**

11. L-arginine is converted into nitric oxide and L-citruline by the enzyme nitric oxide hydroxylase.
Ans. **False.** The enzyme nitric oxide synthetase does this.

12. Both demethylated and didemethylated metabolites of escitalopram are active.
Ans. **True.**

13. Medication-induced movement disorders should be coded on Axis I DSM-IV.
Ans. **True.**

14. Benzodiazepine receptor binding can be inhibited by large doses of caffeine.
Ans. **True.**

15. Amisulpride has been associated with ketoacidosis.
Ans. **False.**

16. Naloxone antagonism of diamorphine at opioid receptors is an example of 'competitive antagonism'.
Ans. **True.**

17. Clozapine should not be used with propylthiouracil.
Ans. **True.**

18. Parkinsonian tremors are finer and faster than non-parkinsonian tremors.
Ans. **False.** The opposite is true.

19. **Risperidone does not affect the pharmacokinetic parameters of lithium.**
Ans. True.

20. **Bromocriptine increases the plasma levels of growth hormone.**
Ans. False. It lowers it.

21. **Coadministration of lithium and metronidazole increases risk of lithium toxicity.**
Ans. True.

22. **Sodium valproate inhibits metabolism of phenytoin, carbamazepine and ethosuximide.**
Ans. True.

23. **Pharmacokinetic interactions alter the plasma concentrations of the interacting drugs.**
Ans. True.

24. **Treatment with olanzapine is associated with increased risk of dyslipidemia.**
Ans. True.

25. **Coadministration of omeprazole and escitalopram can result in reduced plasma concentrations of escitalopram.**
Ans. False. It leads to elevated levels as CYP2C19 is inhibited by omeprazole.

26. **Neuroleptic-induced acute akathisia typically occurs within 4 weeks of initiating or increasing the dose of a neuroleptic medication.**
Ans. True.

27. **Propranolol increases plasma concentration of chlorpromazine.**
Ans. True.

28. **Sulpiride has a low affinity for dopamine receptors in the tubero infundibular tract.**
Ans. False. It has a high affinity. Results in galactorrhoea.

29. **Antiphospholipid antibodies are associated with phenothiazines (e.g. chlorpromazine) in some patients.**
Ans. True.

30. **In functional antagonism two different agonists evoke opposing responses from a single biological system by activating different receptors.**
Ans. True.

31. **Bioavailability of mirtazapine is decreased by more than 50% when coadministered with cimetidine.**
Ans. False. It is increased by >50%.

32. **Tissue tolerance to a drug is different from its metabolic tolerance.**
Ans. True.

33. **Up to two-thirds of depressed patients have a blunted thyrotropin (TSH) response to thyrotropin-releasing hormone (TRH).**
Ans. True.

34. **M-chlorophenylpiperazine is an inactive metabolite of trazodone.**
Ans. False. It is active.

35. **Tamoxifen (an oestrogen receptor antagonist used for the treatment of breast cancer) can induce depression.**
Ans. True.

36. **Lithium-induced fine postural tremor has a frequency between 8 and 12 cycles per second.**
Ans. True.

37. **Gabapentin does not have either active or inactive metabolites.**
Ans. True. It is eliminated unchanged in the urine.

38. The second-generation H$_1$ antagonist astemizole can cause prolongation of the QTc interval, resulting in polymorphic ventricular tachycardia (torsades de pointes).

Ans. **True.**

39. Low serum protein can result in greater sensitivity to conventional doses of lithium.

Ans. **False.** Lithium is not protein-bound.

40. Neuroleptic-induced parkinsonian tremor is a coarse, rhythmic, resting tremor with a frequency between 3 and 6 cycles per second.

Ans. **True.**

41. Benzodiazepine antagonists have no intrinsic activity themselves.

Ans. **True.**

42. Lamotrigine does not affect the metabolism of other drugs.

Ans. **True.**

43. Decreased prolactin levels may be seen following cocaine withdrawal.

Ans. **False.** Elevated prolactin levels may be seen.

44. Clozapine can decrease platelet count.

Ans. **True.**

45. Severe agitation can cause myoglobunuria secondary to muscle breakdown.

Ans. **True.**

46. Risk of cardiac side effects due to tricyclic antidepressants is low when they are coadminstered with Type I antiarrhythmic drugs.

Ans. **False.** The risk is high.

47. Neuroleptic-induced acute dystonia occurs most commonly in young males.

Ans. **True.**

48. The demethyl metabolite of mirtazapine is pharmacologically inactive.

Ans. **False.** It is active.

49. Inverse benzodiazepine agonists decrease the chloride channel openings and produce anxiety and convulsions.

Ans. **True.**

50. Increased levels of serum salicylate can cause organic hallucinosis.

Ans. **True.**

Paper 18

	True	False
1. Leukocytosis is associated with both lithium and neuroleptic malignant syndrome.	☐	☐
2. Lithium induced tremor is usually absent at rest and worsens during intentional movement.	☐	☐
3. Abrupt discontinuation of amantadine may worsen parkinsonism, regardless of the patient's response to therapy.	☐	☐
4. Trazodone has high affinity for muscarinic cholinergic receptors.	☐	☐
5. Inhibition of at least 80 percent of platelet monoamine oxidase activity by MAOI is recommended for antidepressant effect.	☐	☐
6. Carbamazepine can cause a syndrome of inappropriate antidiuretic hormone secretion.	☐	☐
7. In Stage 1 of the human sexual response, libido can be reduced by epinephrine and dopamine reuptake inhibitor (NDRI) bupropion.	☐	☐
8. Both risperidone and 9-hydroxyrisperidone are excreted in human breast milk.	☐	☐
9. Carbamazepine can decrease platelet count.	☐	☐
10. Hypernatremia is associated with increased sensitivity to conventional doses of lithium.	☐	☐
11. Clomipramine has shown efficacy in the treatment of OCD which is independent of its antidepressant effects.	☐	☐
12. A specific polymorphism of the gene encoding dopamine receptor D3 has been associated with increased risk of tardive dyskinesia.	☐	☐
13. Liothyronine has shown efficacy as an augmentation treatment in patients with refractory depression.	☐	☐
14. Serotonin stimulates prolactin release.	☐	☐
15. Toxic reactions to lithium within therapeutic serum levels are not possible.	☐	☐
16. Following an overdose of tricyclic antidepressants their absorption increases.	☐	☐
17. Extreme muscle rigidity in NMS contributes to elevations in creatine kinase.	☐	☐
18. Naloxone is a pure narcotic antagonist with no respiratory depressant effects.	☐	☐
19. The relapse rates of chronic schizophrenic patients have been shown to reduce with drug holidays.	☐	☐
20. The onset of response to an SSRI is slower in depression than in OCD.	☐	☐
21. An association between increased risk of tardive dyskinesia and a polymorphism of the gene encoding the CYP1A2 enzyme has been reported.	☐	☐
22. Water deprivation increases renal lithium clearance.	☐	☐
23. Patients with organic brain syndromes show a higher prevalence rate for TD than those with schizophrenia.	☐	☐
24. Tardive dyskinesia disappears during sleep.	☐	☐

25. Response to an SSRI is usually less robust in depression than in OCD. ☐ ☐

26. The serum prolactin concentration is normal in unmedicated patients with schizophrenia. ☐ ☐

27. Tricyclic antidepressants increase the refractory period and decrease cardiac conduction velocity. ☐ ☐

28. Anticholinergic drugs increase the risk of developing tardive dyskinesia. ☐ ☐

29. Abrupt withdrawal of propanolol can cause rebound tachycardia. ☐ ☐

30. Transdermal oestrogen can improve post natal depression. ☐ ☐

31. In the treatment of OCD, therapeutic effects of behavioural therapy may last longer after stopping treatment than the therapeutic effects of SSRIs after they are stopped. ☐ ☐

32. Medications whose metabolism is by an enzyme with known genetic polymorphisms that affect the rate of metabolism are less likely to be associated with adverse drug reactions. ☐ ☐

33. Hyoscine hydrobromide is effective in treating clozapine-induced hypersalivation. ☐ ☐

34. Antidepressants improve depression before improving psychomotor activity. ☐ ☐

35. Dose of an SSRI should not be increased till steady state is reached. ☐ ☐

36. Prolactin may remain elevated for up to two weeks after cessation of oral antipsychotic treatment and up to six months after cessation of depot antipsychotic treatment. ☐ ☐

37. Serotonin syndrome may progress to rhabdomyolysis. ☐ ☐

38. Lithium is more effective in augmenting antidepressants in unipolar than in bipolar depression. ☐ ☐

39. Drugs with a smaller relative molecular mass are absorbed at a slower rate when they are administered intramuscularly. ☐ ☐

40. Drugs with anticholinergic properties affect verbal memory by impeding semantic organization at encoding. ☐ ☐

41. Theophylline increases lithium clearance. ☐ ☐

42. SSRIs may worsen extrapyramidal effects when given early in the course of antipsychotic therapy. ☐ ☐

43. Hyperprolactinaemia is a recognised side effect of amoxapine. ☐ ☐

44. Antidepressants are ineffective in the elderly depressed patients in the presence of long standing physical illnesses. ☐ ☐

45. Naltrexone aids in preventing relapse in detoxified formerly opioid-dependent patients. ☐ ☐

46. Memantine is licensed for treating mild Alzheimer's disease. ☐ ☐

47. Perimenopausal depression can improve with transdermal oestrogen. ☐ ☐

48. SSRIs cause tachycardia more frequently than they cause bradycardia. ☐ ☐

49. **Bromocriptine acts on presynaptic autoreceptors to inhibit dopaminergic transmission at lower doses and acts as a dopamine postsynaptic receptor agonist at high doses.** ☐ ☐

50. **Sexual side effects are more common with agomelatin than with SSRIs.** ☐ ☐

1. Leukocytosis is associated with both lithium and neuroleptic malignant syndrome.
Ans. True.

2. Lithium induced tremor is usually absent at rest and worsens during intentional movement.
Ans. True.

3. Abrupt discontinuation of amantadine may worsen parkinsonism, regardless of the patient's response to therapy.
Ans. True.

4. Trazodone has high affinity for muscarinic cholinergic receptors.
Ans. False. It has a low affinity.

5. Inhibition of at least 80 percent of platelet monoamine oxidase activity by MAOI is recommended for antidepressant effect.
Ans. True.

6. Carbamazepine can cause a syndrome of inappropriate antidiuretic hormone secretion.
Ans. True.

7. In Stage 1 of the human sexual response, libido can be reduced by epinephrine and dopamine reuptake inhibitor (NDRI) bupropion.
Ans. False. This enhances libido.

8. Both risperidone and 9-hydroxyrisperidone are excreted in human breast milk.
Ans. True.

9. Carbamazepine can decrease platelet count.
Ans. True.

10. Hypernatremia is associated with increased sensitivity to conventional doses of lithium.
Ans. False. Hyponatraemia is associated with this.

11. Clomipramine has shown efficacy in the treatment of OCD which is independent of its antidepressant effects.
Ans. True.

12. A specific polymorphism of the gene encoding dopamine receptor D3 has been associated with increased risk of tardive dyskinesia.
Ans. True.

13. Liothyronine has shown efficacy as an augmentation treatment in patients with refractory depression.
Ans. True.

14. Serotonin stimulates prolactin release.
Ans. True.

15. Toxic reactions to lithium within therapeutic serum levels are not possible.
Ans. False.

16. Following an overdose of tricyclic antidepressants their absorption increases.
Ans. False. It decreases.

17. Extreme muscle rigidity in NMS contributes to elevations in creatine kinase.
Ans. True.

18. Naloxone is a pure narcotic antagonist with no respiratory depressant effects.
Ans. True.

19. The relapse rates of chronic schizophrenic patients have been shown to reduce with drug holidays.

Ans. **False.** They increase.

20. The onset of response to an SSRI is slower in depression than in OCD.

Ans. **False.** The opposite is true.

21. An association between increased risk of tardive dyskinesia and a polymorphism of the gene encoding the CYP1A2 enzyme has been reported.

Ans. **True.**

22. Water deprivation increases renal lithium clearance.

Ans. **False.** It reduces it.

23. Patients with organic brain syndromes show a higher prevalence rate for TD than those with schizophrenia.

Ans. **True.**

24. Tardive dyskinesia disappears during sleep.

Ans. **True.**

25. Response to an SSRI is usually less robust in depression than in OCD.

Ans. **False.** The opposite is true.

26. The serum prolactin concentration is normal in unmedicated patients with schizophrenia.

Ans. **True.**

27. Tricyclic antidepressants increase the refractory period and decrease cardiac conduction velocity.

Ans. **True.**

28. Anticholinergic drugs increase the risk of developing tardive dyskinesia.

Ans. **True.**

29. Abrupt withdrawal of propanolol can cause rebound tachycardia.

Ans. **True.**

30. Transdermal oestrogen can improve post natal depression.

Ans. **True.**

31. In the treatment of OCD, therapeutic effects of behavioural therapy may last longer after stopping treatment than the therapeutic effects of SSRIs after they are stopped.

Ans. **True.**

32. Medications whose metabolism is by an enzyme with known genetic polymorphisms that affect the rate of metabolism are less likely to be associated with adverse drug reactions.

Ans. **False.** The opposite is true.

33. Hyoscine hydrobromide is effective in treating clozapine-induced hypersalivation.

Ans. **True.**

34. Antidepressants improve depression before improving psychomotor activity.

Ans. **False.** The opposite is true.

35. Dose of an SSRI should not be increased till steady state is reached.

Ans. **True.**

36. Prolactin may remain elevated for up to two weeks after cessation of oral antipsychotic treatment and up to six months after cessation of depot antipsychotic treatment.

Ans. **True.**

37. Serotonin syndrome may progress to rhabdomyolysis.

Ans. **True.**

38. **Lithium is more effective in augmenting antidepressants in unipolar than in bipolar depression.**

Ans. **False.** It is more effective in bipolar depression.

39. **Drugs with a smaller relative molecular mass are absorbed at a slower rate when they are administered intramuscularly.**

Ans. **False.** They are aborbed at an increased rate.

40. **Drugs with anticholinergic properties affect verbal memory by impeding semantic organization at encoding.**

Ans. **True.**

41. **Theophylline increases lithium clearance.**

Ans. **True.**

42. **SSRIs may worsen extrapyramidal effects when given early in the course of antipsychotic therapy.**

Ans. **True.**

43. **Hyperprolactinaemia is a recognised side effect of amoxapine.**

Ans. **True.**

44. **Antidepressants are ineffective in the elderly depressed patients in the presence of long standing physical illnesses.**

Ans. **False.**

45. **Naltrexone aids in preventing relapse in detoxified formerly opioid-dependent patients.**

Ans. **True.**

46. **Memantine is licensed for treating mild Alzheimer's disease.**

Ans. **False.** It is licensed for moderate to severe Alzheimer's disease.

47. **Perimenopausal depression can improve with transdermal oestrogen.**

Ans. **True.**

48. **SSRIs cause tachycardia more frequently than they cause bradycardia.**

Ans. **False.** The opposite is true.

49. **Bromocriptine acts on presynaptic autoreceptors to inhibit dopaminergic transmission at lower doses and acts as a dopamine postsynaptic receptor agonist at high doses.**

Ans. **True.**

50. **Sexual side effects are more common with agomelatin than with SSRIs.**

Ans. **False.** Rare.

Paper 19

		True	False
1.	Highly protein bound drugs show higher volume of distribution.	☐	☐
2.	Oestrogen may have antiamyloid properties.	☐	☐
3.	Galantamine has nicotinic receptor agonist properties.	☐	☐
4.	Quetiapine is not associated with increases in serum prolactin levels across its full dose range.	☐	☐
5.	Nausea and vomiting due to SSRIs decrease over time due to gradual desensitization of 5-HT$_2$ receptors.	☐	☐
6.	Chronic antidepressant treatments have been shown to reduce both the proinflammatory cytokines and prostaglandin E2.	☐	☐
7.	Cloned receptors are useful in drug design.	☐	☐
8.	Plasma levels of psychostimulants used in the treatment of ADHD are directly correlated with their therapeutic effects.	☐	☐
9.	Sodium valproate does not act as a microsomal enzyme inducer.	☐	☐
10.	Same dose of a given drug can show a wide inter individual variation in blood levels.	☐	☐
11.	Lithium is metabolized more by hepatic phase I biotransformation than by phase II biotransformation.	☐	☐
12.	Fat to lean body mass ratio is increased in the elderly.	☐	☐
13.	Changing formulations of some drugs can lead to change in the steady-state drug concentrations.	☐	☐
14.	Demethylation of tertiary amine antidepressants to the less toxic secondary amines is faster in the elderly patients.	☐	☐
15.	Low doses of benzodiazepines increase low-voltage fast activity on the EEG.	☐	☐
16.	Clozapine induced agrunlocytosis is more associated with HLA types B38 and DR4.	☐	☐
17.	Antipsychotic induced dystonia is commonest in young females.	☐	☐
18.	SSRIs may induce hypomania or mania in up to 2% of patients with a history of bipolar affective disorder.	☐	☐
19.	SPECT imaging uses radioactively labelled drugs to provide measures of in vivo pharmacology.	☐	☐
20.	Renal clearance of lithium is lower in children and adolescents than in adults.	☐	☐
21.	Lamotrigine acts as a glutamate antagonist by blocking NMDA receptors.	☐	☐
22.	Laboratory findings in neuroleptic malignant syndrome include low serum iron.	☐	☐
23.	Active placebo is a totally inactive tablet.	☐	☐
24.	Antipsychotic drugs decrease levels of neurotensin.	☐	☐
25.	SSRIs are absorbed and metabolized more slowly in children than in adults.	☐	☐

26. Rebound increase in body growth occurs once treatment with psychostimulant drugs in ADHD is discontinued. ☐ ☐

27. Amoxapine is contraindicated in Parkinsonian patients with depression. ☐ ☐

28. Cerebellar signs are seen in serotonin syndrome but not in lithium toxicity. ☐ ☐

29. Stimulant drugs used in the treatment of ADHD enhance performance on tasks requiring fine motor co-ordination and vigilance. ☐ ☐

30. Concurrent use of benzodiazepines with cognitive-behaviour therapy for patients with anxiety disorders is not contraindicated. ☐ ☐

31. Lithium inhibits brain glycogen synthase kinase – 3. ☐ ☐

32. Vigabatrin is an irreversible inhibitor of GABA transaminase. ☐ ☐

33. Antidepressant drugs with high anticholinergic potency are preferable for uncatheterized patients with neurogenic bladder. ☐ ☐

34. Tolerance to Parkinsonian side-effects of antipsychotics can develop. ☐ ☐

35. Theophylline has been associated with prolonged seizure following administration of ECT. ☐ ☐

36. Buspirone is more sedative than the benzodiazepines. ☐ ☐

37. Concentration of phenytoin in the body does not increase proportionately with increases in dosage. ☐ ☐

38. MAO present in platelets and kidney is mainly MAO-A. ☐ ☐

39. Lithium induced hypothyroidism may initiate rapid cycling in some patients with bipolar disorder. ☐ ☐

40. EEG changes with benzodiazepines are more obvious in the parietal regions. ☐ ☐

41. Severe muscular rigidity is seen in neuroleptic malignant syndrome but not in serotonin syndrome. ☐ ☐

42. Depressed mood predicts a good response to stimulant treatment of ADHD. ☐ ☐

43. Benzodiazepines interfere with episodic memory. ☐ ☐

44. MAOIs are contraindicated in patients with carcinoid and pheochromocytoma. ☐ ☐

45. Tolerance to sedation by benzodiazepines takes longer than their tolerance to psychomotor impairment. ☐ ☐

46. For a drug that is always effective the NNT is 1. ☐ ☐

47. Benzodiazepines are useful in the treatment of post-ECT delirium. ☐ ☐

48. Drug induced blockade of 5-HT-2C and H_1 receptors in combination leads to weight gain. ☐ ☐

49. Non-compliance with treatment is included in ICD-10 as a condition that may be a focus of clinical attention. ☐ ☐

50. Placebo is the equivalent of giving no treatment at all. ☐ ☐

Paper 19

1. **Highly protein bound drugs show higher volume of distribution.**
Ans. **False.** They show lower volume of distribution.

2. **Oestrogen may have antiamyloid properties.**
Ans. **True.**

3. **Galantamine has nicotinic receptor agonist properties.**
Ans. **True.**

4. **Quetiapine is not associated with increases in serum prolactin levels across its full dose range.**
Ans. **True.**

5. **Nausea and vomiting due to SSRIs decrease over time due to gradual desensitization of $5-HT_2$ receptors.**
Ans. **False.** This is due to $5-HT_3$ receptors.

6. **Chronic antidepressant treatments have been shown to reduce both the proinflammatory cytokines and prostaglandin E2.**
Ans. **True.**

7. **Cloned receptors are useful in drug design.**
Ans. **True.**

8. **Plasma levels of psychostimulants used in the treatment of ADHD are directly correlated with their therapeutic effects.**
Ans. **False.**

9. **Sodium valproate does not act as a microsomal enzyme inducer.**
Ans. **True.**

10. **Same dose of a given drug can show a wide inter individual variation in blood levels.**
Ans. **True.**

11. **Lithium is metabolized more by hepatic phase I biotransformation than by phase II biotransformation.**
Ans. **False.** Lithium is not metabolized.

12. **Fat to lean body mass ratio is increased in the elderly.**
Ans. **True.**

13. **Changing formulations of some drugs can lead to change in the steady-state drug concentrations.**
Ans. **True.** This is due to differences in the bioavailability of the preparations.

14. **Demethylation of tertiary amine antidepressants to the less toxic secondary amines is faster in the elderly patients.**
Ans. **False.** It is slower in the elderly.

15. **Low doses of benzodiazepines increase low-voltage fast activity on the EEG.**
Ans. **True.**

16. **Clozapine induced agrunlocytosis is more associated with HLA types B38 and DR4.**
Ans. **True.**

17. **Antipsychotic induced dystonia is commonest in young females.**
Ans. **False.** It is more common in young males.

18. **SSRIs may induce hypomania or mania in up to 2% of patients with a history of bipolar affective disorder.**
Ans. **False.** This occurs in up to 20-30% of patients.

19. SPECT imaging uses radioactively labelled drugs to provide measures of in vivo pharmacology.

Ans. True.

20. Renal clearance of lithium is lower in children and adolescents than in adults.

Ans. False. It is higher in children.

21. Lamotrigine acts as a glutamate antagonist by blocking NMDA receptors.

Ans. True.

22. Laboratory findings in neuroleptic malignant syndrome include low serum iron.

Ans. True.

23. Active placebo is a totally inactive tablet.

Ans. False.

24. Antipsychotic drugs decrease levels of neurotensin.

Ans. False. They increase them.

25. SSRIs are absorbed and metabolized more slowly in children than in adults.

Ans. False. This happens more quickly in children.

26. Rebound increase in body growth occurs once treatment with psychostimulant drugs in ADHD is discontinued.

Ans. True.

27. Amoxapine is contraindicated in Parkinsonian patients with depression.

Ans. True. This is because it can produce EPS.

28. Cerebellar signs are seen in serotonin syndrome but not in lithium toxicity.

Ans. False. The opposite is true.

29. Stimulant drugs used in the treatment of ADHD enhance performance on tasks requiring fine motor co-ordination and vigilance.

Ans. True.

30. Concurrent use of benzodiazepines with cognitive-behaviour therapy for patients with anxiety disorders is not contraindicated.

Ans. True.

31. Lithium inhibits brain glycogen synthase kinase – 3.

Ans. True.

32. Vigabatrin is an irreversible inhibitor of GABA transaminase.

Ans. True.

33. Antidepressant drugs with high anticholinergic potency are preferable for uncatheterized patients with neurogenic bladder.

Ans. False. This is true for drugs with low anticholingeric potency.

34. Tolerance to Parkinsonian side-effects of antipsychotics can develop.

Ans. True.

35. Theophylline has been associated with prolonged seizure following administration of ECT.

Ans. True.

36. Buspirone is more sedative than the benzodiazepines.

Ans. False. It is less sedative.

37. Concentration of phenytoin in the body does not increase proportionately with increases in dosage.

Ans. True.

38. **MAO present in platelets and kidney is mainly MAO-A.**

Ans. **False.** It is mainly MAO-B.

39. **Lithium induced hypothyroidism may initiate rapid cycling in some patients with bipolar disorder.**

Ans. **True.**

40. **EEG changes with benzodiazepines are more obvious in the parietal regions.**

Ans. **False.** They are more obvious in the frontal regions.

41. **Severe muscular rigidity is seen in neuroleptic malignant syndrome but not in serotonin syndrome.**

Ans. **True.**

42. **Depressed mood predicts a good response to stimulant treatment of ADHD.**

Ans. **False.**

43. **Benzodiazepines interfere with episodic memory.**

Ans. **True.**

44. **MAOIs are contraindicated in patients with carcinoid and pheochromocytoma.**

Ans. **True.**

45. **Tolerance to sedation by benzodiazepines takes longer than their tolerance to psychomotor impairment.**

Ans. **False.** The opposite is true.

46. **For a drug that is always effective the NNT is 1.**

Ans. **True.**

47. **Benzodiazepines are useful in the treatment of post-ECT delirium.**

Ans. **True.**

48. **Drug induced blockade of 5-HT-2C and H$_1$ receptors in combination leads to weight gain.**

Ans. **True.**

49. **Non-compliance with treatment is included in ICD-10 as a condition that may be a focus of clinical attention.**

Ans. **False.** It is included in DSM-IV but not in ICD-10.

50. **Placebo is the equivalent of giving no treatment at all.**

Ans. **False.**

Paper 20

Questions

	True	False
1. Hydrazine MAOIs can cause reversible peripheral neuropathy.	☐	☐
2. Lithium treatment has been associated with decreased automaticity of SA node.	☐	☐
3. The use of long-acting benzodiazepines in children can impair learning during the daytime.	☐	☐
4. Neuroleptics enhance conditioned avoidance responding to aversive stimuli.	☐	☐
5. β-blockers are effective in reducing SSRI-induced akathisia.	☐	☐
6. Reduced mesenteric blood flow in the elderly can contribute to a decrease in the bioavailability of a drug taken orally.	☐	☐
7. MAOI induced hypertensive crisis due to ingestion of tyramine can be treated with intravenous phentolamine.	☐	☐
8. Patients who are compliant with placebo have shown better outcomes in many disorders than compliant patients treated with an active drug.	☐	☐
9. Drug-induced catalepsy is specific to antipsychotic drugs.	☐	☐
10. Verapamil has shown efficacy as an adjunctive drug in combination with lithium in treatment of bipolar disorder.	☐	☐
11. Conjugation of a drug with glucuronic acid is significantly reduced in the elderly.	☐	☐
12. Lithium levels are increased by angiotensin-converting enzyme (ACE) inhibitors.	☐	☐
13. Stimulant induced hypertension is more common in children of African-Caribbean origin.	☐	☐
14. The addition of psychoeducational family therapy to antipsychotic medication has no effect on the relapse rate of patients with schizophrenia.	☐	☐
15. Topiramate has been associated with kidney stones.	☐	☐
16. In the elderly it is preferable to use benzodiazepines which are metabolised by conjugation than those which are metabolised by hydroxylation and demethylation.	☐	☐
17. The side effects of SSRIs include anxiety.	☐	☐
18. Switching from one class of MAOIs to another can be done immediately.	☐	☐
19. Benzodiazepine-induced ataxia is mediated in the cerebellum.	☐	☐
20. Resistance to taking medication may be related to issues of transference but not counter transference.	☐	☐
21. Coadministration of lithium and metronidazole results in elevated plasma lithium levels.	☐	☐
22. CYP2D6 activity decreases in the elderly.	☐	☐
23. Treatment-resistant depression occurs in one-third of elderly depressed patients.	☐	☐
24. Thrombocytopenia may occur during treatment with sodium valproate.	☐	☐

		True	False
25.	Hydrazine MAOIs are safer for depressed patients with liver disease.	☐	☐
26.	Lithium treatment can cause delayed conduction through the AV node.	☐	☐
27.	Zaleplon shortens sleep onset without prolonging total sleep time.	☐	☐
28.	Patients who respond to placebo have characteristic personality traits.	☐	☐
29.	Studies of the combination of medication and psychotherapy in the maintenance phase of recurring major depressive disorder have shown superiority of combined treatment.	☐	☐
30.	Inhibitory effect of neuroleptics on 'conditioned avoidance responding' shows tolerance with repeated neuroleptic administration.	☐	☐
31.	Binding of a ligand for dopamine transporters shows age-related decline.	☐	☐
32.	The times required for a drug to reach its steady-state therapeutic levels are shorter in the elderly.	☐	☐
33.	Fluoxetine decreases plasma levels of co-administered carbamazepine.	☐	☐
34.	Benzodiazepines may cause anterograde amnesia.	☐	☐
35.	Sertraline has a high risk of causing seizures.	☐	☐
36.	Phenytoin can cause an increase in the mean red corpuscular volume.	☐	☐
37.	Fluoxetine at a dose of 60 mg/day is effective in bulimia nervosa, but not at 20 mg/day.	☐	☐
38.	Lithium reduces slow wave sleep.	☐	☐
39.	Exacerbation of Parkinsonian symptoms has been reported with olanzapine in patients with Parkinson's disease.	☐	☐
40.	In premenopausal females compared with males, gastric emptying is slower, resulting in lower peak blood levels of a drug in females compared with males.	☐	☐
41.	Acamprosate has an antagonistic effect at the NMDA receptor.	☐	☐
42.	'Prokinetic drugs' enhance gastrointestinal transit time and increase the absorption rate.	☐	☐
43.	Benzodiazepines do not affect avoidance in the treatment of PTSD.	☐	☐
44.	Lithium clearance decreases by 30% – 50% during the second half of pregnancy.	☐	☐
45.	Hypothermia and cyanosis are recognised features of floppy infant syndrome due to maternal diazepam use.	☐	☐
46.	The hypothalamus is not protected by blood-brain-barrier.	☐	☐
47.	Urinary retention due to anti Parkinsonian drugs can be reversed by bethanechol.	☐	☐
48.	Benzodiazepines are used to produce pre-operative sedation with amnesia.	☐	☐
49.	The rate of oxidation of alcohol is dependent on the degree of tolerance of the individual.	☐	☐
50.	Iproniazid was originally developed as an antidepressant drug for dysthymia.	☐	☐

1. **Hydrazine MAOIs can cause reversible peripheral neuropathy.**
Ans. **True.**

2. **Lithium treatment has been associated with decreased automaticity of SA node**
Ans. **True.**

3. **The use of long-acting benzodiazepines in children can impair learning during the daytime.**
Ans. **True.**

4. **Neuroleptics enhance conditioned avoidance responding to aversive stimuli.**
Ans. **False.** They inhibit this.

5. **β-blockers are effective in reducing SSRI-induced akathisia.**
Ans. **True.**

6. **Reduced mesenteric blood flow in the elderly can contribute to a decrease in the bioavailability of a drug taken orally.**
Ans. **True.**

7. **MAOI induced hypertensive crisis due to ingestion of tyramine can be treated with intravenous phentolamine.**
Ans. **True.**

8. **Patients who are compliant with placebo have shown better outcomes in many disorders than compliant patients treated with an active drug.**
Ans. **True.**

9. **Drug-induced catalepsy is specific to antipsychotic drugs.**
Ans. **False.**

10. **Verapamil has shown efficacy as an adjunctive drug in combination with lithium in treatment of bipolar disorder.**
Ans. **True.**

11. **Conjugation of a drug with glucuronic acid is significantly reduced in the elderly.**
Ans. **False.** Relatively unaffected.

12. **Lithium levels are increased by angiotensin-converting enzyme (ACE) inhibitors.**
Ans. **True.**

13. **Stimulant induced hypertension is more common in children of African-Caribbean origin.**
Ans. **True.**

14. **The addition of psychoeducational family therapy to antipsychotic medication has no effect on the relapse rate of patients with schizophrenia.**
Ans. **False.** It reduces the relapse rates.

15. **Topiramate has been associated with kidney stones.**
Ans. **True.**

16. **In the elderly it is preferable to use benzodiazepines which are metabolised by conjugation than those which are metabolised by hydroxylation and demethylation.**
Ans. **True.**

17. **The side effects of SSRIs include anxiety.**
Ans. **True.**

18. **Switching from one class of MAOIs to another can be done immediately.**

Ans. **False.** A week gap between two treatment is preferable.

19. **Benzodiazepine-induced ataxia is mediated in the cerebellum.**

Ans. **True.**

20. **Resistance to taking medication may be related to issues of transference but not counter transference.**

Ans. **False.** It may be related to both.

21. **Coadministration of lithium and metronidazole results in elevated plasma lithium levels.**

Ans. **True.**

22. **CYP2D6 activity decreases in the elderly.**

Ans. **False.** It does not change with age.

23. **Treatment-resistant depression occurs in one-third of elderly depressed patients.**

Ans. **True.**

24. **Thrombocytopenia may occur during treatment with sodium valproate.**

Ans. **True.**

25. **Hydrazine MAOIs are safer for depressed patients with liver disease.**

Ans. **False.** Nonhydrazine MAOIs are safer for such patients.

26. **Lithium treatment can cause delayed conduction through the AV node.**

Ans. **True.**

27. **Zaleplon shortens sleep onset without prolonging total sleep time.**

Ans. **True.**

28. **Patients who respond to placebo have characteristic personality traits.**

Ans. **False.**

29. **Studies of the combination of medication and psychotherapy in the maintenance phase of recurring major depressive disorder have shown superiority of combined treatment.**

Ans. **True.**

30. **Inhibitory effect of neuroleptics on 'conditioned avoidance responding' shows tolerance with repeated neuroleptic administration.**

Ans. **True.**

31. **Binding of a ligand for dopamine transporters shows age-related decline.**

Ans. **True.**

32. **The times required for a drug to reach its steady-state therapeutic levels are shorter in the elderly.**

Ans. **False.** It is longer in the elderly.

33. **Fluoxetine decreases plasma levels of co-administered carbamazepine.**

Ans. **False.** It increases this.

34. **Benzodiazepines may cause anterograde amnesia.**

Ans. **True.**

35. **Sertraline has a high risk of causing seizures.**

Ans. **False.**

36. **Phenytoin can cause an increase in the mean red corpuscular volume.**

Ans. **True.**

37. **Fluoxetine at a dose of 60 mg/day is effective in bulimia nervosa, but not at 20 mg/day.**

Ans. **True.**

38. **Lithium reduces slow wave sleep.**

Ans. **False.** It causes an increase to this.

39. **Exacerbation of Parkinsonian symptoms has been reported with olanzapine in patients with Parkinson's disease.**

Ans. **True.**

40. **In premenopausal females compared with males, gastric emptying is slower, resulting in lower peak blood levels of a drug in females compared with males.**

Ans. **True.**

41. **Acamprosate has an antagonistic effect at the NMDA receptor.**

Ans. **True.**

42. **'Prokinetic drugs' enhance gastrointestinal transit time and increase the absorption rate.**

Ans. **True.**

43. **Benzodiazepines do not affect avoidance in the treatment of PTSD.**

Ans. **True.**

44. **Lithium clearance decreases by 30% – 50% during the second half of pregnancy.**

Ans. **False.** It increases at this time.

45. **Hypothermia and cyanosis are recognised features of floppy infant syndrome due to maternal diazepam use.**

Ans. **True.**

46. **The hypothalamus is not protected by blood-brain-barrier.**

Ans. **True.**

47. **Urinary retention due to anti Parkinsonian drugs can be reversed by bethanechol.**

Ans. **True.** Because bethanechol is parasympathomimetic.

48. **Benzodiazepines are used to produce pre-operative sedation with amnesia.**

Ans. **True.**

49. **The rate of oxidation of alcohol is dependent on the degree of tolerance of the individual.**

Ans. **True.**

50. **Iproniazid was originally developed as an antidepressant drug for dysthymia.**

Ans. **False.** It developed as an antitubercular drug.

Paper 21

		True	False
1.	Active transport of a drug can move it up a concentration gradient.	☐	☐
2.	Propranolol has significant effects on neuroleptic induced rigidity.	☐	☐
3.	Acetylcholinesterase inhibitors alter the course of the dementia in the short term.	☐	☐
4.	Carbidopa does not penetrate the blood-brain-barrier.	☐	☐
5.	The norepinephrine transporter gene (SLC6A2) is located on the long arm of chromosome 10.	☐	☐
6.	The dose of a drug required to achieve a specified response is called its 'potency'.	☐	☐
7.	Midazolam is a water soluble benzodiazepine.	☐	☐
8.	Receptors that alter the production of second messengers are called ionotropic receptors.	☐	☐
9.	Dose-response curve can shift left as a result of normal tolerance.	☐	☐
10.	Glucuronidation is always associated with loss of biological activity.	☐	☐
11.	Chlorpromazine can cause pharmacokinetic tolerance.	☐	☐
12.	Cocaine reduces REM sleep and increases REM latency.	☐	☐
13.	Studies have shown that women respond to tricyclic antidepressants such as imipramine better than men respond.	☐	☐
14.	SSRIs are effective in acute treatment of depression but not in relapse prevention.	☐	☐
15.	Reverse tolerance is defined as an increase in potency following chronic exposure to a drug.	☐	☐
16.	Paroxetine reduces plasma levels of procyclidine.	☐	☐
17.	Diazepam increases stage 2, and decreases stages 1 and 4, and REM sleep.	☐	☐
18.	Anxiolytic drugs infused into the amygdalae of animals are known to prevent the acquisition of the conditioned-fear response.	☐	☐
19.	Tricyclic antidepressants may cause REM behaviour disorder.	☐	☐
20.	Olanzapine is effective in treatment of acute agitation associated with bipolar 1 mania.	☐	☐
21.	The diffusion of a drug into the brain is inversely proportional to its water solubility.	☐	☐
22.	An indirect-acting antagonist can reduce the action of a neurotransmitter by depleting its presynaptic stores.	☐	☐
23.	Pharmacokinetic tolerance to benzodiazepines does not exist.	☐	☐
24.	Antimuscarinic action of a drug increases the tendency to develop depolarization blockade.	☐	☐
25.	Blood alcohol level is significantly higher in alcohol-sensitive individuals than in nonsensitive ones.	☐	☐
26.	Acamprosate reduces the effect of excitatory amino acids.	☐	☐

27. Mirtazapine induced side effects include significant sexual dysfunction. ☐ ☐

28. Cocaine shows reverse tolerance following its continued use. ☐ ☐

29. Noradrenergic reuptake inhibitors show significant efficacy in treatment of OCD. ☐ ☐

30. Drugs that either inhibit or induce hepatic CYP450 enzymes cause pharmaco dynamic interactions. ☐ ☐

31. Flumazenil has a shorter half-life than diazepam. ☐ ☐

32. Nicotine has been reported to reduce attentional impairment in adult ADHD. ☐ ☐

33. High protein meals rich in large neutral aminoacids reduces the amount of levodopa that enters the brain. ☐ ☐

34. Log-dose response curves are plotted against the percent maximal response on x-axis. ☐ ☐

35. Morphine activates the Edinger-Westphal nucleus of the oculomotor nerve through μ_2 receptors. ☐ ☐

36. Short-acting hypnotics are better for patients with frequent or early-morning wakening. ☐ ☐

37. A study involving a drug treatment may have a statistically significant result without a clinically significant result. ☐ ☐

38. Tachyphylaxis is defined as a very rapid reduction in the potency of a drug following acute exposure to a drug. ☐ ☐

39. Tardive dyskinesia improves on treatment with procyclidine. ☐ ☐

40. Risk of relapse is higher and sooner after drug discontinuation in depression than in OCD. ☐ ☐

41. Risk of cardiac side effects is higher with aripiprazole than with clozapine. ☐ ☐

42. Side-effects of medication are included in Health of the Nation Outcome Scale (HONOS). ☐ ☐

43. Controlled trials, without randomization, overestimate the benefits of new treatments by 40%. ☐ ☐

44. A direct-acting agonist has both affinity and efficacy at a receptor. ☐ ☐

45. Cerebrospinal fluid concentrations of lithium are higher than those of plasma. ☐ ☐

46. Benzodiazepines can cause pharmacodynamic interactions but not pharmacokinetic interactions. ☐ ☐

47. Prophylactic antipsychotic use improves the outcome in patients with multi-episode schizophrenia. ☐ ☐

48. Every patient who was originally randomized to one or other treatment contributes to the results in 'intention-to-treat analysis'. ☐ ☐

49. Weight gain is a common side-effect of SSRIs. ☐ ☐

50. Hydrolysis is the most common form of drug metabolism. ☐ ☐

Paper 21

1. **Active transport of a drug can move it up a concentration gradient.**
Ans. **True.**

2. **Propranolol has significant effects on neuroleptic induced rigidity.**
Ans. **False.** It does however improve tremor and akathisia.

3. **Acetylcholinesterase inhibitors alter the course of the dementia in the short term.**
Ans. **True.**

4. **Carbidopa does not penetrate the blood-brain-barrier.**
Ans. **True.**

5. **The norepinephrine transporter gene (SLC6A2) is located on the long arm of chromosome 10.**
Ans. **False.** Chromosome 16 at 16q12.2.

6. **The dose of a drug required to achieve a specified response is called its 'potency'.**
Ans. **True.**

7. **Midazolam is a water soluble benzodiazepine.**
Ans. **True.**

8. **Receptors that alter the production of second messengers are called ionotropic receptors.**
Ans. **False.** They are called metabotropic receptors.

9. **Dose-response curve can shift left as a result of normal tolerance.**
Ans. **False.** This happens as a result of reverse tolerance.

10. **Glucuronidation is always associated with loss of biological activity.**
Ans. **True.**

11. **Chlorpromazine can cause pharmacokinetic tolerance.**
Ans. **True.**

12. **Cocaine reduces REM sleep and increases REM latency.**
Ans. **True.**

13. **Studies have shown that women respond to tricyclic antidepressants such as imipramine better than men respond.**
Ans. **False.** Men respond better than women.

14. **SSRIs are effective in acute treatment of depression but not in relapse prevention.**
Ans. **False.** They are effective in both.

15. **Reverse tolerance is defined as an increase in potency following chronic exposure to a drug.**
Ans. **True.**

16. **Paroxetine reduces plasma levels of procyclidine.**
Ans. **False.** It increases procyclidine levels by 40%.

17. **Diazepam increases stage 2, and decreases stages 1 and 4, and REM sleep.**
Ans. **True.**

18. **Anxiolytic drugs infused into the amygdalae of animals are known to prevent the acquisition of the conditioned-fear response.**
Ans. **True.**

19. **Tricyclic antidepressants may cause REM behaviour disorder.**
Ans. **True.**

20. Olanzapine is effective in treatment of acute agitation associated with bipolar 1 mania.
Ans. True.

21. The diffusion of a drug into the brain is inversely proportional to its water solubility.
Ans. True. This is due to the blood-brain-barrier.

22. An indirect-acting antagonist can reduce the action of a neurotransmitter by depleting its presynaptic stores.
Ans. True.

23. Pharmacokinetic tolerance to benzodiazepines does not exist.
Ans. True.

24. Antimuscarinic action of a drug increases the tendency to develop depolarization blockade.
Ans. False. It reduces this tendency.

25. Blood alcohol level is significantly higher in alcohol-sensitive individuals than in nonsensitive ones.
Ans. False. The blood acetaldehyde levels differ.

26. Acamprosate reduces the effect of excitatory amino acids.
Ans. True.

27. Mirtazapine induced side effects include significant sexual dysfunction.
Ans. False.

28. Cocaine shows reverse tolerance following its continued use.
Ans. True.

29. Noradrenergic reuptake inhibitors show significant efficacy in treatment of OCD.
Ans. False.

30. Drugs that either inhibit or induce hepatic CYP450 enzymes cause pharmaco dynamic interactions.
Ans. False. They cause pharmacokinetic interactions.

31. Flumazenil has a shorter half-life than diazepam.
Ans. True.

32. Nicotine has been reported to reduce attentional impairment in adult ADHD.
Ans. True.

33. High protein meals rich in large neutral aminoacids reduces the amount of levodopa that enters the brain.
Ans. True.

34. Log-dose response curves are plotted against the percent maximal response on x-axis.
Ans. False.

35. Morphine activates the Edinger-Westphal nucleus of the oculomotor nerve through μ_2 receptors.
Ans. True.

36. Short-acting hypnotics are better for patients with frequent or early-morning wakening.
Ans. False. Long-acting hypnotics are better for such patients.

37. A study involving a drug treatment may have a statistically significant result without a clinically significant result.
Ans. True.

38. Tachyphylaxis is defined as a very rapid reduction in the potency of a drug following acute exposure to a drug.
Ans. True. It is also known as a rapid tolerance.

39. **Tardive dyskinesia improves on treatment with procyclidine.**

Ans. **False.** It is exacerbated by procyclidine.

40. **Risk of relapse is higher and sooner after drug discontinuation in depression than in OCD.**

Ans. **False.** The opposite is true.

41. **Risk of cardiac side effects is higher with aripiprazole than with clozapine.**

Ans. **False.** Clozapine carries a higher risk.

42. **Side-effects of medication are included in Health of the Nation Outcome Scale (HONOS).**

Ans. **True.** Item No: 5.

43. **Controlled trials, without randomization, overestimate the benefits of new treatments by 40%.**

Ans. **True.**

44. **A direct-acting agonist has both affinity and efficacy at a receptor.**

Ans. **True.**

45. **Cerebrospinal fluid concentrations of lithium are higher than those of plasma.**

Ans. **False.** They are lower.

46. **Benzodiazepines can cause pharmacodynamic interactions but not pharmacokinetic interactions.**

Ans. **True.**

47. **Prophylactic antipsychotic use improves the outcome in patients with multi-episode schizophrenia.**

Ans. **True.**

48. **Every patient who was originally randomized to one or other treatment contributes to the results in 'intention-to-treat analysis'.**

Ans. **True.**

49. **Weight gain is a common side-effect of SSRIs.**

Ans. **False.**

50. **Hydrolysis is the most common form of drug metabolism.**

Ans. **False.** Oxidation is.

Paper 22

	True	False
1. SSRI drugs have no effect on release of 5HT from the presynaptic neurone.	☐	☐
2. The relative potencies of different drugs are determined by comparing their ED_{50} values.	☐	☐
3. The dose-response curve shifts to the left when an agonist is administered in the presence of an antagonist.	☐	☐
4. Buprenorphine is a partial agonist at the μ receptor.	☐	☐
5. Benzodiazepines can be used as substitutes for antidepressants in the treatment of major depression.	☐	☐
6. Desmethylclomipramine is an active metabolite of clomipramine.	☐	☐
7. Antidepressants lose their efficacy over time.	☐	☐
8. A direct-acting antagonist has affinity for a receptor but does not have efficacy at a receptor.	☐	☐
9. β-carbolines are diazepam-binding inhibitors.	☐	☐
10. Direct competition at receptor sites between two drugs may lead to pharmacokinetic interactions.	☐	☐
11. NICE guidance on the use of atypical antipsychotic drugs allows the prescription of atypicals and typicals together when switching.	☐	☐
12. Barnes Akathisia Rating Scale (BAS) covers both subjective and objective aspects of akathisia.	☐	☐
13. Drugs diffuse into the brain in their ionized forms.	☐	☐
14. Lithium, a monovalent cation, diffuses readily into the brain.	☐	☐
15. Both upregulation and down-regulation of a receptor can lead to pharmacodynamic tolerance.	☐	☐
16. Dose-response curve of a drug can shift to right as a result of normal tolerance.	☐	☐
17. Sertraline causes more anticholinergic effects than imipramine.	☐	☐
18. Peripheral neuropathy is a recognised side-effect of MAOIs.	☐	☐
19. Lithium levels are increased by non-steroidal anti-inflammatory drugs.	☐	☐
20. Caffeinism leads to skeletal muscle relaxation.	☐	☐
21. Response to clozapine is correlated with increased ACTH response to m-chlorophenylpiperazine (MCPP).	☐	☐
22. Antipsychotic drugs have been associated with the production of polyclonal IgM autoantibodies.	☐	☐
23. MAOIs can interact with serotonergic drugs to cause serotonin syndrome.	☐	☐
24. Lofepramine can cause more sedation than mirtazapine.	☐	☐

Questions

25. Secondary negative symptoms can be caused by antipsychotic drugs. ☐ ☐

26. Premature ejaculation is a recognised side effect of SSRIs. ☐ ☐

27. Risperidone is a potent LSD antagonist. ☐ ☐

28. All types of tolerance to a drug imply reduction in its potency except behavioural tolerance. ☐ ☐

29. Trazodone causes less sedation than reboxetine. ☐ ☐

30. The dopamine transporter gene (SLC6A3) is located on the short arm of chromosome 5 at 5p15.3. ☐ ☐

31. The threshold for response to clozapine is mostly in the range between 350 μg/L and 600 μg/L. ☐ ☐

32. Men are more likely than women to use prescribed psychotropic drugs. ☐ ☐

33. Norepinephrine antagonism was found with clozapine at doses below those required for apomorphine antagonism. ☐ ☐

34. Risperidone shows curvilinear dose-efficacy relationship. ☐ ☐

35. Venlafaxine has less anticholinergic effects than amitriptyline. ☐ ☐

36. Benzodiazepines have been shown to be effective in treating prodromal symptoms of psychotic relapse. ☐ ☐

37. Discontinuation symptoms following abrupt withdrawal of antipsychotic drugs are symptoms of relapse. ☐ ☐

38. Randomized treatment allocation in clinical trials controls bias. ☐ ☐

39. Clozapine causes moderate increase in seizure threshold. ☐ ☐

40. Highly protein bound drugs will diffuse into the brain slowly. ☐ ☐

41. Lithium therapy increases the activity of protein kinase C. ☐ ☐

42. Benzodiazepine withdrawal is associated with a false-positive result on dexamethasone-suppression test. ☐ ☐

43. Oxcarbazepine does not produce the epoxide metabolite. ☐ ☐

44. A minimum of 4 weeks of treatment with SSRIs is required to evaluate treatment response in OCD. ☐ ☐

45. Clozapine blocks NMDA-antagonist induced electrophysiologic responses. ☐ ☐

46. Nephrotic syndrome is a rare side effect of lithium. ☐ ☐

47. Stimulant drugs are recommended for Kleine-Levin syndrome (KLS). ☐ ☐

48. Neurotransmitters are considered as first messengers. ☐ ☐

49. Prenatal lithium treatment can cause congenital downward displacement of the tricuspid valve into the right ventricle in offspring. ☐ ☐

50. L-tryptophan given before bedtime increases sleep latency. ☐ ☐

Paper 22

1. **SSRI drugs have no effect on release of 5HT from the presynaptic neurone.**
Ans. **True.**

2. **The relative potencies of different drugs are determined by comparing their ED_{50} values.**
Ans. **True.**

3. **The dose-response curve shifts to the left when an agonist is administered in the presence of an antagonist.**
Ans. **False.** It shifts to the right.

4. **Buprenorphine is a partial agonist at the μ receptor.**
Ans. **True.**

5. **Benzodiazepines can be used as substitutes for antidepressants in the treatment of major depression.**
Ans. **False.** They can be used as adjuncts to antidepressants for brief periods.

6. **Desmethylclomipramine is an active metabolite of clomipramine.**
Ans. **True.**

7. **Antidepressants lose their efficacy over time.**
Ans. **False.**

8. **A direct-acting antagonist has affinity for a receptor but does not have efficacy at a receptor.**
Ans. **True.**

9. **β-carbolines are diazepam-binding inhibitors.**
Ans. **True.**

10. **Direct competition at receptor sites between two drugs may lead to pharmacokinetic interactions.**
Ans. **False.** It leads to pharmacodynamic interactions.

11. **NICE guidance on the use of atypical antipsychotic drugs allows the prescription of atypicals and typicals together when switching.**
Ans. **True.**

12. **Barnes Akathisia Rating Scale (BAS) covers both subjective and objective aspects of akathisia.**
Ans. **True.**

13. **Drugs diffuse into the brain in their ionized forms.**
Ans. **False.** They diffuse in their non-ionized forms.

14. **Lithium, a monovalent cation, diffuses readily into the brain.**
Ans. **True.** This is because the molecule is small.

15. **Both upregulation and down-regulation of a receptor can lead to pharmacodynamic tolerance.**
Ans. **True.**

16. **Dose-response curve of a drug can shift to right as a result of normal tolerance.**
Ans. **True.**

17. **Sertraline causes more anticholinergic effects than imipramine.**
Ans. **False.** The opposite is true.

18. **Peripheral neuropathy is a recognised side-effect of MAOIs.**
Ans. **True.**

19. **Lithium levels are increased by non-steroidal anti-inflammatory drugs.**
Ans. **True.**

20. **Caffeinism leads to skeletal muscle relaxation.**
Ans. **False.** It leads to muscle tension.

21. **Response to clozapine is correlated with increased ACTH response to m-chlorophenylpiperazine (MCPP).**
Ans. **True.**

22. **Antipsychotic drugs have been associated with the production of polyclonal IgM autoantibodies.**
Ans. **True.**

23. **MAOIs can interact with serotonergic drugs to cause serotonin syndrome.**
Ans. **True.**

24. **Lofepramine can cause more sedation than mirtazapine.**
Ans. **False.** The opposite is true.

25. **Secondary negative symptoms can be caused by antipsychotic drugs.**
Ans. **True.**

26. **Premature ejaculation is a recognised side effect of SSRIs.**
Ans. **False.** Delayed ejaculation is a side-effect.

27. **Risperidone is a potent LSD antagonist.**
Ans. **True.**

28. **All types of tolerance to a drug imply reduction in its potency except behavioural tolerance.**
Ans. **False.** Reverse tolerance.

29. **Trazodone causes less sedation than reboxetine.**
Ans. **False.** It causes more sedation.

30. **The dopamine transporter gene (SLC6A3) is located on the short arm of chromosome 5 at 5p15.3.**
Ans. **True.**

31. **The threshold for response to clozapine is mostly in the range between 350 μg/L and 600 μg/L.**
Ans. **True.**

32. **Men are more likely than women to use prescribed psychotropic drugs.**
Ans. **False.** Less likely.

33. **Norepinephrine antagonism was found with clozapine at doses below those required for apomorphine antagonism.**
Ans. **True.**

34. **Risperidone shows curvilinear dose-efficacy relationship.**
Ans. **True.**

35. **Venlafaxine has less anticholinergic effects than amitriptyline.**
Ans. **True.**

36. **Benzodiazepines have been shown to be effective in treating prodromal symptoms of psychotic relapse.**
Ans. **True.**

37. **Discontinuation symptoms following abrupt withdrawal of antipsychotic drugs are symptoms of relapse.**
Ans. **False.**

38. **Randomized treatment allocation in clinical trials controls bias.**
Ans. **False.** It controls confounding results.

39. **Clozapine causes moderate increase in seizure threshold.**
Ans. **False.** It reduces seizure threshold.

40. **Highly protein bound drugs will diffuse into the brain slowly.**
Ans. **True.**

41. **Lithium therapy increases the activity of protein kinase C.**
Ans. **False.** It reduces this.

42. **Benzodiazepine withdrawal is associated with a false-positive result on dexamethasone-suppression test.**
Ans. **True.**

43. **Oxcarbazepine does not produce the epoxide metabolite.**
Ans. **True.**

44. **A minimum of 4 weeks of treatment with SSRIs is required to evaluate treatment response in OCD.**
Ans. **False.** A minimum of 12 weeks is required.

45. **Clozapine blocks NMDA-antagonist induced electrophysiologic responses.**
Ans. **True.**

46. **Nephrotic syndrome is a rare side effect of lithium.**
Ans. **True.**

47. **Stimulant drugs are recommended for Kleine-Levin syndrome (KLS).**
Ans. **False.** KLS is self-limiting.

48. **Neurotransmitters are considered as first messengers.**
Ans. **True.**

49. **Prenatal lithium treatment can cause congenital downward displacement of the tricuspid valve into the right ventricle in offspring.**
Ans. **True.**

50. **L-tryptophan given before bedtime increases sleep latency.**
Ans. **False.** It decreases this.

Paper 23

	True	False
1. Approximately 67% of depressed patients fail to respond to placebo treatment.	☐	☐
2. Behavioural disinhibition can be caused by combined use of alcohol and benzodiazepines.	☐	☐
3. Neuroimaging studies have shown hippocampal atrophy under stress leading to depression.	☐	☐
4. Resistance to taking medication may be related to issues of transference and counter transference.	☐	☐
5. A normal serum prolactin can indicate non-compliance with some antipsychotic drugs.	☐	☐
6. Carbamazepine can cause fetal vitamin K deficiency.	☐	☐
7. Poor sleep and appetite are the first symptoms to improve with antidepressant medication after the depressed mood and hopelessness improve.	☐	☐
8. Side effects of valproate include hair loss.	☐	☐
9. Incidence of rash may be increased with use of lamotrigine with valproate.	☐	☐
10. The sensitivity of central benzodiazepine receptors is studied by measuring the velocity of the saccadic eye movements.	☐	☐
11. Failure to respond to one acetylcholinesterase inhibitor means that the patient will not respond to another.	☐	☐
12. Calcium ion is a second messenger.	☐	☐
13. Placebo-induced analgesia may be blocked by naloxone.	☐	☐
14. Patients who are in remission from their depression may be considered asymptomatic unlike those who are responders to the medication but not yet in remission.	☐	☐
15. Ziprasidone causes more weight gain than zotepine.	☐	☐
16. The half-life values of the tricyclic antidepressants are greater in the elderly.	☐	☐
17. Phenothiazines are known to cause elevated total bilirubin and direct bilirubin values.	☐	☐
18. Outcome with pharmacological treatments in OCD is good in the presence of compulsive behaviour.	☐	☐
19. Heterocyclic antidepressants with serotoninergic reuptake inhibition effect are effective in the treatment of panic disorder.	☐	☐
20. Patients with Bipolar I disorder are at reduced risk of developing rapid cycling with the use of tricyclic antidepressants.	☐	☐
21. Depressed patients with two or more prior episodes need maintenance antidepressant therapy.	☐	☐
22. Pentagastrin is an agonist of the type B cholecystokinin receptor.	☐	☐

23. The half-life of an MAOI is shorter in slow acetylators. ☐ ☐

24. Neuroreceptor imaging has helped to establish the optimal dosage range of antipsychotic drugs. ☐ ☐

25. Repression of the gene for brain-derived neurotrophic factor (BDNF) under stress has been implicated in the causation of depression. ☐ ☐

26. Adenylate cyclase is an intracellular enzyme. ☐ ☐

27. Mianserin can be used for a depressed patient who is on clozapine. ☐ ☐

28. Renal clearance of a drug increases towards the end of pregnancy. ☐ ☐

29. Phencyclidine acts as an agonist of the NMDA subtype of glutamate receptor. ☐ ☐

30. 5% to 10% of patients with OCD may not respond to treatment with SSRIs. ☐ ☐

31. Response to lithium is likely to be poor in the absence of a family history of bipolar I disorder. ☐ ☐

32. Antidepressant medication reduces the relapse rates more in the first year following successful initial treatment than in the later years. ☐ ☐

33. More than 50% of the monoamines released from the nerve terminal are catabolized by catechol-O-methyltransferase. ☐ ☐

34. Desmethyldiazepam has been described as an endogenous anxiolytic ligand. ☐ ☐

35. Stereoisomers of a drug have different molecular formulae. ☐ ☐

36. Nocebo phenomenon refers to the development of adverse effects due to placebo. ☐ ☐

37. NMDA-antagonists induce schizophrenia-like symptoms. ☐ ☐

38. L-tryptophan deficient diet can decrease the risk of relapse in depressed patients who are on serotonergic antidepressants. ☐ ☐

39. Sensitivity of platelet and lymphocyte benzodiazepine receptors is high in generalized anxiety disorder. ☐ ☐

40. Dopamine synthesizing enzymes include tyrosine hydroxylase. ☐ ☐

41. Genetic differences in hepatic metabolism contribute significantly to the large interindividual variation in the metabolism of antidepressants. ☐ ☐

42. Plasma prolactin levels are decreased with ECT. ☐ ☐

43. The therapeutic index for lithium is quite low. ☐ ☐

44. Carbamazepine has been associated with false-negative results on the dexamethasone suppression test. ☐ ☐

45. Valproate can cause thrombocytopenia. ☐ ☐

46. Depressed patients can be switched into hypomanic or manic episodes by both antidepressant medications and phototherapy. ☐ ☐

47. Cocaine is a weak inhibitor of the dopamine transporter. ☐ ☐

48. **Dale's Law only applies to the presynaptic portion of the neuron.**   ☐   ☐

49. **Increased neutral amino acid intake blocks the entry of L-tryptophan into the brain.**   ☐   ☐

50. **Serine hydroxymethylase is an essential enzyme for the synthesis of glycine.**   ☐   ☐

Paper 23

1. Approximately 67% of depressed patients fail to respond to placebo treatment.
Ans. True.

2. Behavioural disinhibition can be caused by combined use of alcohol and benzodiazepines.
Ans. True.

3. Neuroimaging studies have shown hippocampal atrophy under stress leading to depression.
Ans. True.

4. Resistance to taking medication may be related to issues of transference and counter transference.
Ans. True.

5. A normal serum prolactin can indicate non-compliance with some antipsychotic drugs.
Ans. True.

6. Carbamazepine can cause fetal vitamin K deficiency.
Ans. True.

7. Poor sleep and appetite are the first symptoms to improve with antidepressant medication after the depressed mood and hopelessness improve.
Ans. False. Sleep and appetite improve before other symptoms of depression.

8. Side effects of valproate include hair loss.
Ans. True.

9. Incidence of rash may be increased with use of lamotrigine with valproate.
Ans. True.

10. The sensitivity of central benzodiazepine receptors is studied by measuring the velocity of the saccadic eye movements.
Ans. True.

11. Failure to respond to one acetylcholinesterase inhibitor means that the patient will not respond to another.
Ans. False.

12. Calcium ion is a second messenger.
Ans. True.

13. Placebo-induced analgesia may be blocked by naloxone.
Ans. True.

14. Patients who are in remission from their depression may be considered asymptomatic unlike those who are responders to the medication but not yet in remission.
Ans. True.

15. Ziprasidone causes more weight gain than zotepine.
Ans. False. Zotepine causes more weight gain.

16. The half-life values of the tricyclic antidepressants are greater in the elderly.
Ans. True.

17. Phenothiazines are known to cause elevated total bilirubin and direct bilirubin values.
Ans. True.

18. Outcome with pharmacological treatments in OCD is good in the presence of compulsive behaviour.
Ans. False.

19. **Heterocyclic antidepressants with serotoninergic reuptake inhibition effect are effective in the treatment of panic disorder.**

Ans. **True.** For example, imipramine.

20. **Patients with Bipolar I disorder are at reduced risk of developing rapid cycling with the use of tricyclic antidepressants.**

Ans. **False.** They are at increased risk.

21. **Depressed patients with two or more prior episodes need maintenance antidepressant therapy.**

Ans. **True.**

22. **Pentagastrin is an agonist of the type B cholecystokinin receptor.**

Ans. **True.**

23. **The half-life of an MAOI is shorter in slow acetylators.**

Ans. **False.**

24. **Neuroreceptor imaging has helped to establish the optimal dosage range of antipsychotic drugs.**

Ans. **True.**

25. **Repression of the gene for brain-derived neurotrophic factor (BDNF) under stress has been implicated in the causation of depression.**

Ans. **True.**

26. **Adenylate cyclase is an intracellular enzyme.**

Ans. **True.**

27. **Mianserin can be used for a depressed patient who is on clozapine.**

Ans. **False.** It increases the risk of agranulocytosis.

28. **Renal clearance of a drug increases towards the end of pregnancy.**

Ans. **True.**

29. **Phencyclidine acts as an agonist of the NMDA subtype of glutamate receptor.**

Ans. **False.** It acts as an antagonist.

30. **5% to 10% of patients with OCD may not respond to treatment with SSRIs.**

Ans. **False.** 30% – 50% of such patients may not respond.

31. **Response to lithium is likely to be poor in the absence of a family history of bipolar I disorder.**

Ans. **True.**

32. **Antidepressant medication reduces the relapse rates more in the first year following successful initial treatment than in the later years.**

Ans. **True.**

33. **More than 50% of the monoamines released from the nerve terminal are catabolized by catechol-O-methyltransferase.**

Ans. **False.** Not more than 10%.

34. **Desmethyldiazepam has been described as an endogenous anxiolytic ligand.**

Ans. **True.**

35. **Stereoisomers of a drug have different molecular formulae.**

Ans. **False.**

36. **Nocebo phenomenon refers to the development of adverse effects due to placebo.**

Ans. **True.**

37. **NMDA-antagonists induce schizophrenia-like symptoms.**

Ans. **True.**

38. **L-tryptophan deficient diet can decrease the risk of relapse in depressed patients who are on serotonergic antidepressants.**

Ans. False.

39. **Sensitivity of platelet and lymphocyte benzodiazepine receptors is high in generalized anxiety disorder.**

Ans. False.

40. **Dopamine synthesizing enzymes include tyrosine hydroxylase.**

Ans. True.

41. **Genetic differences in hepatic metabolism contribute significantly to the large interindividual variation in the metabolism of antidepressants.**

Ans. True.

42. **Plasma prolactin levels are decreased with ECT.**

Ans. False. They are increased.

43. **The therapeutic index for lithium is quite low.**

Ans. True.

44. **Carbamazepine has been associated with false-negative results on the dexamethasone suppression test.**

Ans. False. It is associated with false-positive results.

45. **Valproate can cause thrombocytopenia.**

Ans. True.

46. **Depressed patients can be switched into hypomanic or manic episodes by both antidepressant medications and phototherapy.**

Ans. True.

47. **Cocaine is a weak inhibitor of the dopamine transporter.**

Ans. False. It is a strong inhibitor.

48. **Dale's Law only applies to the presynaptic portion of the neuron.**

Ans. True.

49. **Increased neutral amino acid intake blocks the entry of L-tryptophan into the brain.**

Ans. True.

50. **Serine hydroxymethylase is an essential enzyme for the synthesis of glycine.**

Ans. True.

Paper 24

Questions

1. D-cycloserine, a partial agonist at the glycine regulatory site on the NMDA receptor, has shown efficacy in treatment of schizophrenia. ☐ ☐

2. Family psychoeducational therapy is more effective in reducing the relapse rate in schizophrenia when combined with antipsychotic drugs. ☐ ☐

3. Ecstasy acts as an antagonist at 5HT2A receptor sites. ☐ ☐

4. Monoamine oxidase is found both in brain and intestines. ☐ ☐

5. Glutamate's actions are terminated by enzymatic breakdown. ☐ ☐

6. The degree to which the effect of a neuroleptic drug on negative symptoms is mediated by its effects on other symptoms, can be studied by path analysis. ☐ ☐

7. Radiolabels used in neuroreceptor imaging studies give information about the distribution of the drug bound to radio labels. ☐ ☐

8. Yohimbine blocks the effects of α_2–receptor agonists. ☐ ☐

9. Antidepressant efficacy in clinical trials has been shown to be higher than antidepressant effectiveness in reducing relapses in clinical practice. ☐ ☐

10. Depolarization produces opening of voltage-dependent calcium channels. ☐ ☐

11. Lithium induced Ebstein's anomaly can be identified with prenatal screening with a high-resolution ultrasound examination and fetal echocardiography at 16–18 weeks gestation. ☐ ☐

12. An antagonist at presynaptic 5HT1D terminal auto receptor blocks the release of 5HT. ☐ ☐

13. Raised interferon alpha levels in the CSF of children with schizophrenia are correlated with refractoriness to drug treatment. ☐ ☐

14. Neuroleptic-induced deficit syndrome is probably related to blockade of D_2 receptors in the nigrostriatal pathway. ☐ ☐

15. Topiramate is a weak inhibitor of carbonic anhydrase. ☐ ☐

16. Olanzapine blocks NMDA-antagonist induced deficits in prepulse inhibition. ☐ ☐

17. Stevens-Johnson syndrome is a common side effect of carbamazepine. ☐ ☐

18. Dopamine is a precursor of norepinephrine for noradrenergic neurons. ☐ ☐

19. G proteins are present in cell membrane. ☐ ☐

20. Zotepine inhibits norepinephrine reuptake. ☐ ☐

21. The extent of placental passage is lower for olanzapine than for quetiapine. ☐ ☐

22. Risk factors for drug-induced hepatotoxicity include female gender. ☐ ☐

23. Sildenafil should not be prescribed to patients who are on organic nitrates. ☐ ☐

24. High doses of valproate can cause prolonged bleeding time. ☐ ☐

25. Cholinergic muscarinic receptors are metabotropic receptors linked to G proteins. ☐ ☐

	True	False

26. Vitamin E is a weak free-radical scavenger. ☐ ☐

27. Venlafaxine is a weak inhibitor of dopamine reuptake. ☐ ☐

28. The maintenance dose of an SSRI for the treatment of panic disorder is lower than its starting dose. ☐ ☐

29. Changes in hepatic circulation have significant effect on the clearance of drugs. ☐ ☐

30. Sodium valproate is a broad-spectrum antiepileptic drug. ☐ ☐

31. The apolipoprotein E4 allele has been shown to be associated with a good response to cholinesterase inhibitor treatment of Alzheimer's dementia. ☐ ☐

32. Increased urinary pH decreases excretion of weak bases. ☐ ☐

33. Repeated cocaine use can cause reverse tolerance. ☐ ☐

34. The action of neuropeptides is terminated by monoamine oxidase. ☐ ☐

35. The type of neuro transmitter activating heteroceptors differs from that released from the axon. ☐ ☐

36. Lamotrigine reduces the effectiveness of oral contraceptives. ☐ ☐

37. Heteroceptors are activated by neurotransmitters different from those produced by the nerve they are on. ☐ ☐

38. L-α-acetylmethadol (LAAM) is a derivative of methadone with a longer duration of action. ☐ ☐

39. Anandamide is the psychoactive ingredient in marijuana. ☐ ☐

40. Dopamine beta-hydroxylase converts norepinephrine into dopamine. ☐ ☐

41. Phenylketonuria can be caused by tetrahydrobiopterin deficiency. ☐ ☐

42. Lithium has been proposed to deplete intracellular inositol levels resulting in attenuation of phosphoinositide signalling in neurons. ☐ ☐

43. Osmotic diuretics decrease lithium excretion. ☐ ☐

44. Agonists of H_3 receptors augment slow-wave sleep. ☐ ☐

45. Fluoxetine, 20 mg/day has been shown to be as effective as 60 mg/day in treatment of bulimia nervosa. ☐ ☐

46. Among neurotransmitter signals GABA is faster in onset than monoamines or neuropeptides. ☐ ☐

47. Maintenance valproate treatment has shown equal efficacy in reducing the frequency and severity of both manic and depressive episodes. ☐ ☐

48. Clomipramine induced decreases in cerebro-spinal fluid levels of 5-hydroxydole-acetic acid are correlated with improvement in obsessive-compulsive symptoms. ☐ ☐

49. Vigabatrine should not be initiated as monotherapy except in West's syndrome. ☐ ☐

50. Studies have shown increased antidepressant efficacy of SSRI drugs in depressed patients homozygous for the short allele of the serotonin transporter promoter. ☐ ☐

Paper 24

1. D-cycloserine, a partial agonist at the glycine regulatory site on the NMDA receptor, has shown efficacy in treatment of schizophrenia.
Ans. True.

2. Family psychoeducational therapy is more effective in reducing the relapse rate in schizophrenia when combined with antipsychotic drugs.
Ans. True.

3. Ecstasy acts as an antagonist at 5HT2A receptor sites.
Ans. False. It acts as partial agonist.

4. Monoamine oxidase is found both in brain and intestines.
Ans. True.

5. Glutamate's actions are terminated by enzymatic breakdown.
Ans. False. They are terminated via removal by transport pumps.

6. The degree to which the effect of a neuroleptic drug on negative symptoms is mediated by its effects on other symptoms, can be studied by path analysis.
Ans. True.

7. Radiolabels used in neuroreceptor imaging studies give information about the distribution of the drug bound to radio labels.
Ans. True.

8. Yohimbine blocks the effects of α_2–receptor agonists.
Ans. True.

9. Antidepressant efficacy in clinical trials has been shown to be higher than antidepressant effectiveness in reducing relapses in clinical practice.
Ans. False.

10. Depolarization produces opening of voltage-dependent calcium channels.
Ans. True.

11. Lithium induced Ebstein's anomaly can be identified with prenatal screening with a high-resolution ultrasound examination and fetal echocardiography at 16–18 weeks gestation.
Ans. True.

12. An antagonist at presynaptic 5HT1D terminal auto receptor blocks the release of 5HT.
Ans. False. It increases 5HT release.

13. Raised interferon alpha levels in the CSF of children with schizophrenia are correlated with refractoriness to drug treatment.
Ans. True.

14. Neuroleptic-induced deficit syndrome is probably related to blockade of D_2 receptors in the nigrostriatal pathway.
Ans. False. It is probably the mesocortical dopamine pathway.

15. Topiramate is a weak inhibitor of carbonic anhydrase.
Ans. True.

16. Olanzapine blocks NMDA-antagonist induced deficits in prepulse inhibition.
Ans. True.

17. Stevens-Johnson syndrome is a common side effect of carbamazepine.
Ans. False. It is rare.

18. Dopamine is a precursor of norepinephrine for noradrenergic neurons.
Ans. True.

19. G proteins are present in cell membrane.
Ans. True.

20. Zotepine inhibits norepinephrine reuptake.
Ans. True.

21. The extent of placental passage is lower for olanzapine than for quetiapine.
Ans. False. Higher for olanzapine.

22. Risk factors for drug-induced hepatotoxicity include female gender.
Ans. True.

23. Sildenafil should not be prescribed to patients who are on organic nitrates.
Ans. True.

24. High doses of valproate can cause prolonged bleeding time.
Ans. True.

25. Cholinergic muscarinic receptors are metabotropic receptors linked to G proteins.
Ans. True.

26. Vitamin E is a weak free-radical scavenger.
Ans. True.

27. Venlafaxine is a weak inhibitor of dopamine reuptake.
Ans. True.

28. The maintenance dose of an SSRI for the treatment of panic disorder is lower than its starting dose.
Ans. False. It is higher than the starting dose.

29. Changes in hepatic circulation have significant effect on the clearance of drugs.
Ans. True.

30. Sodium valproate is a broad-spectrum antiepileptic drug.
Ans. True.

31. The apolipoprotein E4 allele has been shown to be associated with a good response to cholinesterase inhibitor treatment of Alzheimer's dementia.
Ans. False. It is associated with a poor response.

32. Increased urinary pH decreases excretion of weak bases.
Ans. True.

33. Repeated cocaine use can cause reverse tolerance.
Ans. True.

34. The action of neuropeptides is terminated by monoamine oxidase.
Ans. False. It is by catabolic peptidases.

35. The type of neuro transmitter activating heteroceptors differs from that released from the axon.
Ans. True.

36. Lamotrigine reduces the effectiveness of oral contraceptives.
Ans. False.

37. Heteroceptors are activated by neurotransmitters different from those produced by the nerve they are on.
Ans. True.

38. **L-α-acetylmethadol (LAAM) is a derivative of methadone with a longer duration of action.**

Ans. **True.**

39. **Anandamide is the psychoactive ingredient in marijuana.**

Ans. **False.** Anandamide is an endocannabinoid.

40. **Dopamine beta-hydroxylase converts norepinephrine into dopamine.**

Ans. **False.** It converts dopamine into norepinephrine.

41. **Phenylketonuria can be caused by tetrahydrobiopterin deficiency.**

Ans. **True.**

42. **Lithium has been proposed to deplete intracellular inositol levels resulting in attenuation of phosphoinositide signalling in neurons.**

Ans. **True.**

43. **Osmotic diuretics decrease lithium excretion.**

Ans. **False.** They enhance it.

44. **Agonists of H_3 receptors augment slow-wave sleep.**

Ans. **True.**

45. **Fluoxetine, 20 mg/day has been shown to be as effective as 60 mg/day in treatment of bulimia nervosa.**

Ans. **False.** 60 mg/day is more effective.

46. **Among neurotransmitter signals GABA is faster in onset than monoamines or neuropeptides.**

Ans. **True.**

47. **Maintenance valproate treatment has shown equal efficacy in reducing the frequency and severity of both manic and depressive episodes.**

Ans. **False.** It is less effective in depressive episodes.

48. **Clomipramine induced decreases in cerebro-spinal fluid levels of 5-hydroxydole-acetic acid are correlated with improvement in obsessive-compulsive symptoms.**

Ans. **False.** Positively correlated.

49. **Vigabatrine should not be initiated as monotherapy except in West's syndrome.**

Ans. **True.**

50. **Studies have shown increased antidepressant efficacy of SSRI drugs in depressed patients homozygous for the short allele of the serotonin transporter promoter.**

Ans. **False.** This is true for patients homozygous for the long allele.

Paper 25

1. **Brussel sprouts cause induction of drug metabolism through the induction of:**
A) CYP 1A2
B) CYP 2E1
C) CYP 2D6
D) CYP 3A4
E) CYP 1A9

2. **Factors causing decreasing clearance of a drug include the following except:**
A) Normal variation
B) Old age
C) Renal failure
D) Enzyme induction
E) Liver failure

3. **Following are true about first- order elimination except:**
A) The decline in plasma concentration is not constant with time.
B) It varies with the concentration.
C) Examples include ethanol.
D) The concentration declines exponentially with time.
E) The higher the concentration, the greater the rate of elimination.

4. **Identify the false statement regarding the half-life of a drug**
A) It provides an index of the time-course of drug elimination.
B) It provides an index of the time-course of drug-accumulation.
C) It guides the choice of dose-interval.
D) The smaller the volume of distribution (Vd) the longer the half-life.
E) The larger the clearance (Cl), the shorter the half-life (t1/2).

5. **Identify the Phase II reaction of the drug metabolism from the following:**
A) Desulphuration
B) Hydrolysis
C) Deamination
D) Sulphation
E) Dealkylation

6. **Identify the ion channel-linked first messenger from the following:**
A) Dopamine
B) Norepinephrine
C) Histamine
D) Acetylcholine (muscarinic)
E) Acetylcholine (nicotinic)

7. **Identify the second messenger from the following:**
A) BDNF
B) Activated phosphokinase A
C) GSK-3
D) Inositol triphosphate (IP3)
E) NGF

8. **Targets of direct psychotropic drug action can include the following except:**
A) Monoamine transporters
B) Enzymes
C) Voltage-sensitive ion channels
D) Ligand gated ion channels
E) Genes

9. **Cigarette smoking causes inhibition of one of the following:**
A) CYP 2D6
B) CYP 1A2
C) CYP 3A4
D) CYP 2E1
E) CYP 1D4

10. **Identify the most common haemotological effect of valproate from the following:**
A) Leukocytosis
B) Thrombocytopenia
C) Anaemia
D) Leucopenia
E) Reticulocytosis

11. **Examples of the ligand gate ionotropic receptors include the following except:**
A) GABA A
B) Nicotinic
C) Glycine
D) NMDA
E) Muscarinic

12. **Examples of the metabotropic G-protein coupled receptors include the following except:**
A) Dopaminergic
B) Adrenergic
C) Serotonergic
D) Cannabinoid receptors
E) GABA A

13. **Stereoisomers of a drug may differ from each other in the following except:**
A) Efficacy
B) Safety
C) Order of attachment of atoms
D) Potency
E) Side effects

14. **Identify the false statement:**
A) Partial agonists increase signal transduction in the absence of a full agonist.
B) Antagonists have the opposite action of agonists.
C) Antagonists block the action of agonists.
D) Antagonists have no activity of their own in the absence of agonists.
E) Inverse agonists do have opposite actions compared to agonists.

15. **Identify the false statement from the following:**
A) Vigabatrin inhibits GABA transaminase.
B) Sildenafil inhibits phosphodiesterase.
C) Lithium inhibits phosphatidylinositol.
D) Metronidazole inhibits aldehyde dehydrogenase.
E) Donepezil inhibits butyrylcholinesterase.

16. **Identify the false statement regarding the placebo effect:**
A) It is evident much earlier than the usual response to a drug.
B) More evident in patients with anxiety than in those with schizophrenia.
C) More evident in patients with acute disorders.
D) An 'active placebo' mimics the adverse effects of the drug being studied.
E) It decreases according to patient's expectancy.

17. **Following recovery a single episode of depression should be treated for minimum:**
A) 7 days
B) 2 weeks
C) 2 years
D) 6 months
E) 6 weeks

18. **Lithium is estimated to increase the life-expectancy by:**
A) 2 years
B) 5 years
C) 3 years
D) 7 years
E) 12 years

19. **Steady state level of a drug is achieved after:**
A) 3 half-lives
B) 5 half-lives
C) 7 half-lives
D) 1 half-life
E) 2 half-lives

20. **Licence to market a drug is obtained:**
A) Before phase I
B) Before phase II
C) Before phase III
D) After phase IV
E) After phase III

21. **Identify the correct statement regarding the pharmacokinetics in children:**
A) Bioavailability is higher than in adults.
B) Hepatic drug metabolism is slower than in adults.
C) Protein binding is more than in adults.
D) Drug crosses BBB less readily than in adults.
E) Variation in a drug's metabolism is less than in adults.

22. **Lithium discontinuation leads to recurrence of affective disorder in 3/12 in:**
A) 90% of the patients.
B) 50% of the patients.
C) 10% of the patients.
D) 25% of the patients.
E) 2% of the patients.

23. **Identify the false statement regarding the pharmacokinetics of MAOIs:**
A) The acetylation status is inherited through a single gene.
B) 50% of caucasians are fast acetylators.
C) Extensively metabolised by the liver.
D) Irreversible non-selective MAOIs are highly lipid soluble.
E) They have a long elimination half-life.

24. **Risk factors for dystonia include the following except:**
A) Younger age
B) Drug naïve patient
C) Male gender
D) Slow discontinuation of antipsychotic
E) Rapid escalation in dose

25. **Risk factors for akathisia include the following except:**
A) Lower dosage
B) High potency drug
C) Drug naïve patient
D) Rapid escalation in dose
E) Polypharmacy

26. **Risk factors for parkinsonism include the following except:**
A) High potency antipsychotic
B) Higher dosage
C) Advancing age
D) Male gender
E) Head injury

27. **Risk factors for tardive dyskinesia include the following except:**
A) Male gender
B) Advancing age
C) Dementia
D) EPS
E) Autism

28. **Identify the false statement regarding neuroleptic malignant syndrome (NMS):**
A) Lithium can cause NMS.
B) Symptoms include tachycardia.
C) Metoclopramide can improve NMS.
D) Incidence ranges from 0.15% to 0.07%.
E) Rigidity can be localised.

29. **Identify the false statement regarding NMS:**
A) NMS begins with rigidity.
B) Body temperature rises faster in NMS than in malignant hyperthermia.
C) Myoclonus is common with serotonin syndrome but not in NMS.
D) Muscles are flaccid in heat stroke but not in NMS.
E) NMS has no strong genetic component.

30. **Identify the incorrect statement about antidepressant discontinuation syndrome:**
A) More common with fluoxetine.
B) Paraesthesia is a common symptom.
C) Symptoms rarely start after a week.
D) More common after longer periods of treatment.
E) Psychotic symptoms are not uncommon after stopping MAOI.

31. **Risk factors for torsade de pointes include the following except:**
A) Female gender
B) Hypermagnesemia
C) Hypokalaemia
D) Bradycardia
E) Heart failure

32. **Risk of cardiac arrhythmias is lower with the following group of antipsychotics except:**
A) Substituted benzamide
B) Thienobenzodiazepine
C) Benzisoxazole
D) Dibenzodiazepine
E) Dibenzothiepine

33. **Identify the common cardiovascular adverse effect of antipsychotic drugs:**
A) Ventricular tachycardia
B) Myocarditis
C) Postural hypotension
D) Widened QRS complex
E) Prolongation of the QT interval

34. **Identify the NMDA receptor antagonist from the following antidementia drugs:**
A) Piracetam
B) Donepezil
C) Rivastigmine
D) Memantine
E) Co-dergocrine

35. **Acetycholinesterase inhibitors may exacerbate the following except:**
A) Seizures
B) Bradycardia
C) Atrioventricular block
D) Polyuria
E) Parkinson's disease

36. **The adverse effects of anticholinergic drugs include the following except:**
A) Constipation
B) Dry mouth
C) Confusion
D) Pinpoint pupil
E) Hallucinations

37. **Sudden discontinuation of anticholinergic drugs results in the following except:**
A) Insomnia
B) Salivation
C) Constipation
D) Restlessness
E) Abdominal pain

38. **Identify the false statement regarding anticholinergic drugs:**
A) They impair the therapeutic effects of antipsychotic drugs.
B) They may reduce the risk of developing tardive dyskinesia.
C) They may show euphoriant action.
D) They may have stimulant properties.
E) They improve dystonia better than akathisia.

39. **Following are true about acamprosate except:**
A) It is an agonist at the GABA receptor.
B) It is an antagonist at the glutamate receptor.
C) It is contraindicated with simultaneous use of alcohol.
D) It reduces craving for alcohol.
E) It should be commenced after alcohol withdrawal.

40. **Identify the false statement about methadone:**
A) Half life is approximately 12 hrs.
B) Has high affinity for the mu opioid receptor.
C) It is less sedating than morphine.
D) It should not be administered with MAOIs.
E) Adverse effects include hypothermia.

41. **Following are true about lofexidine except:**
A) It is an α_2 antagonist.
B) It causes less hypotension than clonidine.
C) It prevents withdrawal in opioid dependent patients.
D) It should not be used if the pulse rate is <50/mt.
E) Abrupt discontinuation causes hypertension

42. **Identify the selective CB1 receptor antagonist from the following:**
A) Reserpine
B) Ranitidine
C) Reboxetine
D) Rimonabant
E) Ramelteon

43. **Identify the false statement regarding phosphodiesterase 5 inhibitors:**
A) Effective for the treatment of SSRI induced sexual dysfunction.
B) Should not be coadministered with amylnitrates.
C) Recognised sideeffects include sudden visual loss.
D) Metabolism is predominantly via CYP3A4
E) Tadalafil has shorter half life than sildenafil.

44. **Common sideffects of lamotrigine include the following except:**
A) Diplopia
B) Ataxia
C) Headache
D) Aplastic anaemia
E) Drowsiness

45. **Long acting benzodiazepines include the following except:**
A) Chlordiazepoxide
B) Clonazepam
C) Lormetazepam
D) Clobazam
E) Clorazepate

46. **Features of benzodiazepine withdrawal syndrome include the following except:**
A) Insomnia
B) Myalgia
C) Weight loss
D) Diplopia
E) Paraesthesia

47. **Identify the false statement regarding buspirone:**
A) It has no affinity for the melatonin recptors.
B) Does not alleviate benzodiazepine withdrawal.
C) Not contraindicated in epilepsy.
D) Does not cause cognitive impairment.
E) Does not inhibit dopaminergic activity.

48. **Lithium toxicity can be precipitated by the following except:**
A) Dehydration
B) Impaired renal function
C) CYP2D6 inhibitors
D) Diuretics
E) Severe infection

49. **After stopping MAOIs, their effects last up to:**
A) 4 hrs
B) 12 hrs
C) 4 mths
D) 2 wks
E) 36 hrs

50. **General side-effects of MAOIs include the following except:**
A) Hypotension
B) Dystonia
C) Insomnia
D) Psychomotor arousal
E) May induce manic episode

Paper 25

1. **Brussel sprouts cause induction of drug metabolism through the induction of:**
Ans. **A)** CYP 1A2

2. **Factors causing decreasing clearance of a drug include the following except:**
Ans. **D)** Enzyme induction

3. **Following are true about first- order elimination except:**
Ans. **C)** Examples include ethanol.

4. **Identify the false statement regarding the half-life of a drug**
Ans. **D)** The smaller the volume of distribution (Vd) the longer the half-life.

5. **Identify the Phase II reaction of the drug metabolism from the following:**
Ans. **D)** Sulphation

6. **Identify the ion channel-linked first messenger from the following:**
Ans. **E)** Acetylcholine (nicotinic)

7. **Identify the second messenger from the following:**
Ans. **D)** Inositol triphosphate (IP3)

8. **Targets of direct psychotropic drug action can include the following except:**
Ans. **E)** Genes

9. **Cigarette smoking causes inhibition of one of the following:**
Ans. **B)** CYP 1A2

10. **Identify the most common haemotological effect of valproate from the following:**
Ans. **B)** Thrombocytopenia

11. **Examples of the ligand gate ionotropic receptors include the following except:**
Ans. **E)** Muscarinic

12. **Examples of the metabotropic G-protein coupled receptors include the following except:**
Ans. **E)** GABA A

13. **Stereoisomers of a drug may differ from each other in the following except:**
Ans. **C)** Order of attachment of atoms

14. **Identify the false statement:**
Ans. **B)** Antagonists have the opposite action of agonists.

15. **Identify the false statement from the following:**
Ans. **E)** Donepezil inhibits butyrylcholinesterase.

16. **Identify the false statement regarding the placebo effect:**
Ans. **E)** It decreases according to patient's expectancy.

17. **Following recovery a single episode of depression should be treated for minimum:**
Ans. **E)** 6 weeks

18. **Lithium is estimated to increase the life-expectancy by:**
Ans. **D)** 7 years

19. **Steady state level of a drug is achieved after:**
Ans. **B)** 5 half-lives

20. **Licence to market a drug is obtained:**
Ans. **E)** After phase III

21. **Identify the correct statement regarding the pharmacokinetics in children:**
Ans. **E)** Variation in a drug's metabolism is less than in adults.

22. **Lithium discontinuation leads to recurrence of affective disorder in 3/12 in:**
Ans. **B)** 50% of the patients.

23. **Identify the false statement regarding the pharmacokinetics of MAOIs:**
Ans. **A)** The acetylation status is inherited through a single gene.

24. **Risk factors for dystonia include the following except:**
Ans. **D)** Slow discontinuation of antipsychotic

25. **Risk factors for akathisia include the following except:**
Ans. **A)** Lower dosage

26. **Risk factors for parkinsonism include the following except:**
Ans. **D)** Male gender

27. **Risk factors for tardive dyskinesia include the following except:**
Ans. **E)** Autism

28. **Identify the false statement regarding neuroleptic malignant syndrome (NMS):**
Ans. **C)** Metoclopramide can improve NMS.

29. **Identify the false statement regarding NMS:**
Ans. **B)** Body temperature rises faster in NMS than in malignant hyperthermia.

30. **Identify the incorrect statement about antidepressant discontinuation syndrome:**
Ans. **A)** More common with fluoxetine.

31. **Risk factors for torsade de pointes include the following except:**
Ans. **B)** Hypermagnesemia

32. **Risk of cardiac arrhythmias is lower with the following group of antipsychotics except:**
Ans. **D)** Dibenzodiazepine

33. **Identify the common cardiovascular adverse effect of antipsychotic drugs:**
Ans. **C)** Postural hypotension

34. **Identify the NMDA receptor antagonist from the following antidementia drugs:**
Ans. **D)** Memantine

35. **Acetycholinesterase inhibitors may exacerbate the following except:**
Ans. **D)** Polyuria

36. **The adverse effects of anticholinergic drugs include the following except:**
Ans. **D)** Pinpoint pupil

37. **Sudden discontinuation of anticholinergic drugs results in the following except:**
Ans. **C)** Constipation

38. **Identify the false statement regarding anticholinergic drugs:**
Ans. **B)** They may reduce the risk of developing tardive dyskinesia.

39. **Following are true about acamprosate except:**
Ans. **C)** It is contraindicated with simultaneous use of alcohol.

40. **Identify the false statement about methadone:**
Ans. **A)** Half life is approximately 12 hrs.

41. **Following are true about lofexidine except:**
Ans. **A)** It is an α_2 antagonist.

42. **Identify the selective CB1 receptor antagonist from the following:**
Ans. **D)** Rimonabant

43. **Identify the false statement regarding phosphodiesterase 5 inhibitors:**
Ans. **E)** Tadalafil has shorter half life than sildenafil.

44. **Common sideffects of lamotrigine include the following except:**
Ans. **D)** Aplastic anaemia

45. **Long acting benzodiazepines include the following except:**
Ans. **C)** Lormetazepam

46. **Features of benzodiazepine withdrawal syndrome include the following except:**
Ans. **D)** Diplopia

47. **Identify the false statement regarding buspirone:**
Ans. **C)** Not contraindicated in epilepsy.

48. **Lithium toxicity can be precipitated by the following except:**
Ans. **C)** CYP2D6 inhibitors

49. **After stopping MAOIs, their effects last up to:**
Ans. **D)** 2 wks

50. **General side-effects of MAOIs include the following except:**
Ans. **B)** Dystonia

Paper 26

1. Receptor affinities of antidepressant drugs
   Match up to three options (a – h) with each of the drugs (1 – 3):

a) Monoamine oxidase B
b) The noradrenergic reuptake transporter
c) The alpha 2 receptor
d) The dopamine 2 receptor
e) The dopaminergic reuptake transporter
f) The 5HT2A receptor
g) The 5HT3 receptor
h) The serotonin reuptake tranporter

1) **Tricyclic antidepressants** _____

2) **Mirtazapine** _____

3) **Nefazodone** _____

2. Combination strategies
   Match up to two combination strategies (a – g) with scenarios (1 – 3) below :

a) **Add lithium to antidepressant treatment**
b) **Add buspirone to an SSRI**
c) **Add an atypical antipsychotic drug to an SSRI**
d) **Add amisulpride to reboxetine**
e) **Combine an SSRI and reboxetine**
f) **Combine a tricyclic antidepressant and a benzodiazepine**
g) **Add an atypical antipsychotic to lithium carbonate**

1) **Unipolar depression refractory to monotherapy** _____

2) **Obsessive compulsive disorder refractory to monotherapy** _____

3) **Panic disorder refractory to monotherapy** _____

3. Efficacy/Diagnosis
   Match up to four drugs (a – h) with the conditions (1 – 3) below they are effective in their treatment of:

a) Moclobemide
b) Citalopram
c) Buspirone
d) Propranolol
e) Imipramine
f) Buproprion
g) Clonazepam
h) Clonidine

1) **Panic disorder** _____

2) **Social phobia** _____

3) **Post traumatic stress disorder** _____

4. Adverse effects of antipsychotic drugs

Match up to three side effects (a – h) above with each of the drugs (1 – 3) below:

a) Prolonged QTc interval
b) Neutropenia
c) Type 2 diabetes
d) Nausea
e) Marked weight gain
f) Insomnia
g) Tardive dyskinesia
h) Hyperprolactinaemia

1) Clozapine _____

2) Aripiprazole _____

3) Haloperidol _____

5. Glutamate

Match up to two of (a – h) with each of the processes (1 – 3) below:

a) A presynaptic transporter
b) The sigma site
c) Mitochondrial glutaminase
d) A glial transporter
e) The kainite receptor
f) The NMDA receptor
g) The metabotropic glutamate receptor
h) Dendritic pruning

1) Synthesis of glutamate _____

2) Synaptic removal of glutamate _____

3) Glutamatergic excitotoxicity _____

6. Receptor properties

Match up to three receptor properties (a – h) with the receptors (1 – 3) below:

a) Mediates cortical memory function
b) Allosterically modulated by zinc
c) Ligand gated
d) May be inhibitory
e) Antagonised by scopolamine
f) Antagonised by curare
g) G-protein linked
h) Acts as its own presynaptic transporter

1) The muscarinic receptor _____

2) The nicotinic receptor _____

3) The M1 postsynaptic acetylcholine receptor _____

7. Cholinesterase inhibitors
   Match up to two of options (a – h) above with the drugs (1 – 3) below:

a) Is hepatotoxic
b) Inhibits acetylcholinesterase
c) Inhibits butylcholinesterase
d) Is reversible
e) Is pseudoirreversible
f) Is a prodrug
g) Acts as a nicotinic agonist
h) Permanently halts the manifestations of Alzheimer's disease

1) Donepezil _____

2) Rivastigmine _____

3) Galantamine _____

8. Substance misuse
   Match up to three of (a – g) with the drugs (1 – 3) below:

a) Acts at mu, delta and kappa receptors
b) Releases opiates and endocannabinoids
c) Enhances the actions of the GABA-A receptor complex
d) Reduces NMDA mediated excitation
e) Piloerection occurs in the withdrawal syndrome
f) Anandamide is an endogenous version
g) Acts at CB1 and CB2 receptors

1) Alcohol _____

2) Cannabis _____

3) Opioids _____

9. Sexual functions
   Match up to three of (a – h) above which are involved in sexual functions (1 – 3) below:

a) Anandamide
b) Nitric oxide
c) Serotonin
d) Cholesystokinin
e) Dopamine
f) Prolactin
g) Acetylcholine
h) Noradrenaline

1) Libido _____

2) Arousal and erection _____

3) Orgasm and ejaculation _____

10. CYP450 enzymes

Match up to 2 drugs (a – h) with each effect on CYP450 enzymes (1 – 3) below:

a) Carbamazepine
b) Paroxetine
c) Fluvoxamine
d) Phenytoin
e) Aripiprazole
f) Venlafaxine
g) Clozapine
h) Fluoxetine

1) Inhibition of 3A4 _____

2) Induction of 2C19 _____

3) Inhibition of 2D6 _____

11. Signal transduction cascades

Link the signal transduction cascades (1 – 2) with up to 3 messengers (a – g) below:

a) cAMP
b) GABA-A
c) Nicotinic
d) IP3
e) Protein kinase
f) Ca^{+2}
g) Norepinephrine

1) G – protein linked _____

2) Ion- channel linked _____

12. Drug metabolism enzymes

Link the phases (1 – 2) of drug metabolism with up to 4 appropriate enzymes (a – g) below:

a) N- acetyltransferase
b) CYP2C9
c) CYP2D6
d) Thiopurine methyl tranferase
e) CYP2C19
f) Glutathione –s-transferase
g) Aldehyde dehydrogenase

1) Phase 1 _____

2) Phase 2 _____

13. Presynaptic monoamine transporters

Link the presynaptic monoamine transporters (1 – 3) with up to 4 substrates (a – h) below:

a) Amphetamines
b) Serotonin
c) Ecstacy
d) Epinephrine
e) Dopamine
f) Glutamate
g) Norepinephrine
h) Glycine

1) Dopamine transporter (DAT) ______________________________

2) Serotonin transporter (SERT) ______________________________

3) Norepinephrine transporter (NET) ______________________________

14. Side effects of antiepileptic drugs

Link up to 4 the side effects (a – i) with each of the anti epileptic drugs (1 – 3) below:

a) Diplopia
b) Insomnia
c) Acute pancreatitis
d) Dizziness
e) Tremor
f) Stevens-Johnson syndrome
g) Aplastic anaemia
h) Weight gain
i) Hair loss

1) Lamotrigine ______________________________

2) Sodium valproate ______________________________

3) Carbamazepine ______________________________

15. Drug interactions

Link up to 4 drug combinations (a – g) with each type of drug interactions (1 – 2) below:

a) Diuretics and lithium
b) Flumazenil and diazepam
c) Phenytoin and valproate
d) Alcohol and diazepam
e) SSRI and tricyclics
f) SSRI and MAOI
g) Lithium and SSRI

1) Pharmacodynamic interactions ______________________________

2) Pharmacokinetic interactions ______________________________

Drug metabolites
Match up to 5 of the drugs (a – h) with its type of metabolite (1 – 2) below:

a) Paroxetine
b) Clomipramine
c) Duloxetine
d) Diazepam
e) Carbamazepine
f) Aripiprazole
g) Lamotrigine
h) Trazodone

1) Metabolite is active _____

2) Metabolite is inactive _____

17. Psychotropics in pregnancy
Match each of the 3 scenarios (1 – 3) with up to 3 appropriate clinical actions (a – i) below:

a) Recommended bottle feeds
b) 'Wait and see'
c) Admit to mother and baby unit
d) Switch to sodium valproate
e) Recommend venlafaxine instead
f) Recommend sertraline instead
g) Recommend an atypical antipsychotic instead
h) Consider psychotherapeutic instead
i) Discuss the risks with the patient

1) Twenty year old female with bipolar affective disorder wishing to become pregnant

_____

2) Female with depression on fluoxetine on postnatal day1 who wants to breast feed

_____

3) Breastfeeding mother asking for diazepam for anxiety

_____

18. SSRI profiles
Match up to two of the statements (a – h) with each of the SSRI profiles (1 – 3) below:

a) Affinity for the sigma site is important for this indication
b) The starting dose is higher than for other indications
c) Target symptoms worsen before they improve
d) Response is slower, a trial should last up to six months
e) Response is faster but may be poorly maintained
f) Response is frequently a complete recovery
g) Discontinuation syndrome is more problematic in this indication
h) There is unexplained variation between different exemplars in the same patient

1) SSRIs in depression _____

2) SSRIs in OCD _____

3) SSRIs in bulimia _____

Paper 26

1. Receptor affinities of antidepressant drugs
   Match up to three options (a – h) with each of the drugs (1 – 3)

Ans. 1) b, h
   2) c, f, g
   3) h, f

2. Combination strategies
   Match up to two combination strategies (a – g) with scenarios (1 – 3) below

Ans. 1) a, e
   2) b, c
   3) f, g

3. Efficacy/Diagnosis
   Match up to four drugs (a – h) with the conditions (1 – 3) below they are effective in their treatment of:

Ans. 1) a, b, e, g
   2) a, b, d, g
   3) a, b, e

4. Adverse effects of antipsychotic drugs
   Match up to three side effects (a – h) above with each of the drugs (1 – 3) below

Ans. 1) b, c, e
   2) d, f
   3) g, h

5. Glutamate
   Match up to two of (a – h) with each of the processes (1 – 3) below

Ans. 1) c
   2) a, d
   3) f, h

6. Receptor properties
   Match up to three receptor properties (a – h) with the receptors (1 – 3) below

Ans. 1) d, e, g
   2) c, f
   3) a

7. Cholinesterase inhibitors
   Match up to two of options (a – h) above with the drugs (1 – 3) below

Ans. 1) b, d
   2) b, e
   3) b, g

8. Substance misuse
   Match up to three of (a – g) with the drugs (1 – 3) below

Ans. 1) b, c, d
   2) f, g
   3) a, e

9. Sexual functions
   Match up to three of (a – h) above which are involved in sexual functions (1 – 3) below

Ans. 1) e, f
   2) b, g
   3) c, h

10. CYP450 enzymes

Match up to 2 drugs (a – h) with each effect on CYP450 enzymes (1 – 3) below

Ans. 1) h
2) a
3) b, h

11. Signal transduction cascades

Link the signal transduction cascades (1 – 2) with up to 3 messengers (a – g) below

Ans. 1) a, d, g
2) b, c, f

12. Drug metabolism enzymes

Link the phases (1 – 2) of drug metabolism with up to 4 appropriate enzymes (a – g) below

Ans. 1) b, c, e, g
2) a, d, f

13. Presynaptic monoamine transporters

Link the presynaptic monoamine transporters (1 – 3) with up to 4 substrates (a – h) below:

Ans. 1) a, d, e, g
2) b, c
3) a, d, e, g

14. Side effects of antiepileptic drugs

Link up to 4 the side effects (a – i) with each of the anti epileptic drugs (1 – 3) below:

Ans. 1) b, d, f
2) c, e, h, i
3) a, d, g

15. Drug interactions

Link up to 4 drug combinations (a – g) with each type of drug interactions (1 – 2) below

Ans. 1) b, d, f, g
2) a, c, e

16. Drug metabolites

Match up to 5 of the drugs (a – h) with its type of metabolite (1 – 2) below

Ans. 1) b, d, e, f, h
2) a, c, g

17. Psychotropics in pregnancy

Match each of the 3 scenarios (1 – 3) with up to 3 appropriate clinical actions (a – i) below

Ans. 1) a, g, i
2) f, h, i
3) a, h, i

18. SSRI profiles

Match up to two of the statements (a – h) with each of the SSRI profiles (1 – 3) below

Ans. 1) f
2) d, h
3) b, e

Bibliography

American Psychiatric Association. DSM-IV TR. Diagnostic and Statistical Manual of Mental Disorders. 4th ed. Washington DC: American Psychiatric Association; 2000.

Anderson IM, Reid IC. Fundamentals of Clinical Psychopharmacology. London & New York:Taylor & Francis Group; 2004

Baxter K. Stockley's Drug Interactions. 9th ed. London: Pharmaceutical Press; 2010

Bazire, S. Psychotropic Drug Directory. Aberdeen: Healthcomm UK Ltd; 2010

Begg EJ. Instant Clinical Pharmacology. Oxford: Wiley-Blackwell; 2002

Brunton LL, Lazo JS, Parker KL (eds). Goodman & Gilman's The Pharmacological Basis of Therapeutics. 12th ed. New York, NY: McGraw Hill; 2011

Chee HN, Keh-Ming L, Singh BS, Chiu EY. Ethno-psychopharmacology: Advances in Current Practice (Cambridge Medicine). Cambridge: Cambridge University Press; 2008

Cookson, J, Taylor,D, Katona C. Use of Drugs in Psychiatry. 5th ed. London: Gaskell; 2002

Davies DM, Ferner RE, de Glanville (eds). Davies's Textbook of Adverse Drug Reactions. London: Chapman and Hall Medical; 1999

Davis KL, Charney D, Coyle JT, Nemeroff C (eds). Neuropsychopharmacology. The Fifth Generation of Progress. Philadelphia: Lippincott Williams & Wilkins; 2002

Dhillon S, Kostrzewski A. Clinical Pharmacokinetics. London: Pharmaceutical Press; 2006

Fawcett J, Stein DJ, Jobson KO. Textbook of Treatment Algorithms in Psychopharmacology; New York: John Wiley & Sons; 1999

Gelder M, Andreason N, Lopez-Ibor J, Geddes J. New Oxford Textbook of Psychiatry. Vol 2. Oxford: Oxford University Press; 2009

Gorwood P, Hamon M. Psychopharmacogenetics. London: Springer; 2006

Green WH. Child and Adolescent Psychopharmacology. 4th ed. Philadelphia, PA: Lippincott Williams & Wilkins; 2007

Haddad P, et al. Adverse Syndromes and Psychiatric Drugs – A Clinical Guide. Oxford: OUP; 2005

Jacobson SA, Pies R, Katz IR. Clinical Manual of Geriatric Psychopharmacology. American Psychiatric Publishing; 2007

Joint Formulary Committee. British National Formulary (BNF) 62. 62nd ed. London: Pharmaceutical Press; 2011

Karalliedde K, Henry J (eds). Handbook of Drug Interactions. London: Arnold; 1998

Kruk ZL, Pycock CJ. Neurotransmitters and Drugs. 3rd ed. London: Chapman and Hall; 1991

Kalyna Z, Bezchlibnyk-Butler BJ, Jeffries J. Clinical Handbook of Psychotropic Drugs. 16th ed. Ashland, OH: Hogrefe; 2006

King DJ. Seminars in Clinical Psychiatry. Gaskell; 2004

Lee A. Adverse Drug Reactions. 2nd ed. London: Pharmaceutical Press; 2006

Leonard BE. Fundamentals of Psychopharmacology. 3rd ed. Chichester: Wiley; 2003

Lerer B. Pharmacogenetics of Psychotropic Drugs. New York: Cambridge University Press; 2002

Mrazek DA. Psychiatric Pharmacogenomics. New York: Oxford University Press; 2010

Musa MN (ed). Pharmacokinetics and Therapeutic Monitoring of Psychiatric Drugs. Springfield, Illinois: Charles C Thomas; 1993

Owens DGC. A Guide to the Extrapyramidal Side-effects of Antipsychotic drugs. Cambridge: Cambridge University Press; 1999

Pedro R. Ethnicity and Psychopharmacology (Review of Psychiatry, Vol 19, No. 4). Washington DC: American Psychiatric Press; 2000

Pies RW. Handbook of Essential Psychopharmacology. 2nd edn. New York: Oxford University Press; 2005

Puri BK, Tyre PJ. Sciences Basic to Psychiatry. Edinburgh: Churchill Livingstone; 1992

Rang HP, Dale MM, Ritter JM, Flower RJ. Rang and Dale's Pharmacology. 6th ed. Edinburgh: Churchill Livingstone Elsevier; 2007

Reveley MA, Deakin JFW (eds). The Psychopharmacology of Schizophrenia. London: Arnold Publishers; 2001

Sadock BJ, Sadock VA, Ruiz P. Comprehensive Textbook of Psychiatry, Vol. 2. 9th edn. Philadelphia, PA: Wolters Kluwer Health/Lippincott Williams & Wilkins; 2009

Schatzberg AF, Nemeroff CB (eds). Textbook of Psychopharmacology. 4th edn. Washington DC: American Psychiatric Publishing, Inc; 2009

Schatzberg AF, Cole JO, DeBattista C. Manual of Clinical Psychopharmacology. 7th edn. Washington DC: American Psychiatric Publishing Inc; 2010

Schwab M, Kaschka WP, Spina E. Pharmacogenomics in Psychiatry. Basel: Karger; 2010

Shiloh R, Stryjer R, Nutt D, Weizman A. Atlas of Psychiatric Pharmacotherapy. 2nd ed. London: Informa Healthcare; 2006

Sibley DR., Hanin I, Kuhar M, Skolnick P (eds). Handbook of Contemporary Neuropharmacology. 3 Vols. Hoboken, NJ: Wiley Interscience; 2007

Spiegel R. Psychopharmacology – An Introduction. 4th ed. Chichester: Wiley & Sons; 2003

Stahl SM. Antipsychotics and Mood Stabilizers: Stahl's Essential Psychopharmacology. 3rd edn. New York: Cambridge University Press; 2008

Stahl SM. Essential Psychopharmacology. Neuroscientific basis and Practical Applications. 3rd edn. Cambridge, UK: Cambridge University Press; 2008

Stahl SM. Essential Psychopharmacology: The Prescriber's Guide. Cambridge, UK: Cambridge University Press; 2009

Stein DJ, Lerer B, Stahl SM. Evidence-based Psychopharmacology; Cambridge University Press; 2005

Taylor D, Paton C. Case Studies in Psychopharmacology. 2nd edn. London: Martin Dunitz; 2002

Taylor D, Paton C, Kapur S. The Maudsley Prescribing Guidelines. 10th edn. London: Informa Healthcare; 2009

Tyrer P. Psychopharmacology of Anxiety. Oxford: Oxford University Press; 1989

Walsh BT (ed). Child Psychopharmacology. Washington DC: American Psychiatric Association; 1998

Weber WW. Pharmacogenetics. 2nd edn. Oxford University Press; 2008

World Health Organization. The ICD-10 Classification of Mental and Behavioural Disorders; 1992. WHO website. www.who.int/entity/classifications/icd/en/GRNBOOK.pdf. Accessed 13 Oct 2011.

Wright P. Core Psychopharmacology. In: Wright P, Phelan M, Stern J, eds. Core Psychiatry. 2nd edn. London: Elsevier Saunders; 2006